"Mom . . . I'm pregnant"

"Mom...

"I'm pregnant"

BEV O'BRIEN

TYNDALE HOUSE PUBLISHERS, INC. WHEATON, ILLINOIS

Scripture references throughout, noted
"RSV," were taken from the *Holy Bible,
Revised Standard Version,* copyrighted 1946,
1952; © 1971, 1973, National Council of the
Churches of Christ in the U.S.A., Division of
Education and Ministry; New York.

First printing, August 1982
Library of Congress Catalog Card 82-50437
ISBN 0-8423-4495-0, paper

*I wish to express my
appreciation to my daughter,
for allowing her story to
be told*

*To Mary Brite, whose
encouragement started and
kept me writing*

*And to Manon Strong and others
who helped critique
my manuscript.*

CONTENTS

Introduction

It was early September 1950. On a cold, drizzly afternoon, after a day visiting at Minnesota's Itasca State Park, we were on our way home. Mother was driving.

Suddenly I heard the sound of tires screeching. As I looked up, I realized that the sound came from our car. It swerved back and forth. Just ahead, the road curved sharply to the right.

"I can't turn!" Mother cried out, her voice filled with panic. "I can't stop!"

Immediately I knew we would never make the turn. I opened my mouth to scream, but no sound came out.

Before I had a chance to brace myself, I was tumbling from the car seat to the roof, and finally back to the seat again, all in a tangle of arms and legs with my sister.

I remember my father's reaching over and turning off the ignition. Then we all began to take inventory of ourselves. Miraculously, none of us was hurt. When we climbed out of our crumpled car, it was apparent that we had gone over a steep bank, rolled completely over, and landed right side up.

For weeks after that, I would wake in the middle of

the night, gripped by that sheer, stark terror I had
known when I realized that we were out of control and
powerless to change our situation.

I can never know panic, to this day, without thinking
of that accident. It was the first thing that came to my
mind when I learned that my unmarried nineteen-year-
old daughter was pregnant. Again, I was that terrified,
helpless youngster.

But I couldn't allow myself to give in to panic. I was
the one Sandy turned to for help.

Certain times in a girl's life seem to require the help
and support of another woman, and I was that woman
for Sandy. For another girl, it might be a different
relative, or a teacher, or neighbor, or pastor's wife, or
friend, or even a friend's mother.

However, being chosen to help doesn't necessarily
mean that a woman is at all ready or capable to do so.

I remember my own struggle. First I had to overcome
my own bitter feelings. Then I had to find out what the
real world of the unwed mother consists of today, as
opposed to what I had known when I was Sandy's age.
I had to sort through a jumble of decisions, each
clamoring to be considered first, and separate what only
appeared urgent from what really was.

I needed, too, to acknowledge my limitations as a
helper and, where I wasn't qualified, to help Sandy seek
out professional assistance.

Most important of all, I tried to be an example to
Sandy of true Christian charity, and to be always in
prayer for her and her baby. I wanted to help her to
keep her eyes on future possibilities for her life, not on
past failures.

It was God's mercy and grace that brought me
through that long-ago car accident safely. As I reflect on
Sandy's unwed pregnancy, I see the same merciful and
gracious God in action.

1

Off to Never, Never Land

Sandy had been dragging around for a week, barely able to get from her bed to the couch. She didn't appear to be seriously ill. She just complained of a generalized fatigue and that food tasted funny.

Because she was nineteen, I assumed she could tell me if she needed medical attention. When several more days passed and she still hadn't improved, though, I called our family physician's office. "We can see her tomorrow," the nurse told me.

That Friday afternoon, although in early February, was clear and sunny. I had brought a book to read, so I told Sandy I would wait for her in the car. To my surprise, she was back in less than ten minutes.

"What did he say?"

Sandy closed the car door and stared out of the window. When she spoke, I could barely hear her. "I have to bring in a urine specimen Monday morning. Mom . . . he thinks I'm pregnant."

It seemed an eternity before her answer stopped ringing in my ears. It couldn't be. I couldn't—no, I wouldn't—believe it. Never once had I even remotely considered such a possibility.

Automatically, I began the familiar motions of driving, although later I would remember very little of the trip from physician's office to home.

Inside my head, a thousand thoughts jostled and pushed to gain my attention.

How could she do this to me? She knew better. Of course she did; her father and I had done our best. . . . Her father—how would I ever tell him? He'd really hit the ceiling. And his parents, too. They'd think we had failed. We *had* failed.

And everyone will know it—unless the test comes back negative. Maybe it will. It could. Maybe nobody will have to know about this. Even if she is pregnant, lots of women are having abortions. But, of course, we wouldn't consider that; we don't believe in that. Still, the test might come back negative.

With painful clarity, I recalled the conversation I'd had with a friend only days earlier. What was that I'd said— that I had a lot of confidence in my daughters, and that I'd never have to worry about any of them? Oh, no, how am I ever going to face her? And everyone at church. What are they going to think of Sandy? And of me?

I looked at Sandy, and she seemed to be perfectly calm. Didn't she even care? The idea that she might be pregnant made me sick. I felt as I had the time when she'd come out from swimming with an ugly black leech clinging to the back of her leg. It was repulsive. "Get that thing off you!" I'd shouted.

But this ugly, terrible thing wasn't going to be brushed aside that easily. It was there to stay—if she truly was pregnant.

Once during that drive home Sandy called out to me, "Stop!" At first, I thought that she somehow knew the thoughts that were racing through my mind. Then, as through a deep fog, I realized that she meant for me to stop for the red light I was quickly approaching.

But I couldn't turn off my mind. What would we do with a baby? To whom did we last loan our crib?

A terrible bitterness began to seep through me. I didn't want to talk to Sandy, or even to look at her.

When we finally arrived home, each of us went in a different direction. Sandy headed straight for her room and pulled her door shut behind her. I went to the kitchen.

First I ate several chocolate chip cookies and drank a glass of milk. Then I took out a piece of cheese and a slice of leftover meat loaf and devoured that. (Some people can't eat when they become upset; I can't stop.)

How could I tell Sandy's father? I couldn't begin to think. Then, with relief, I remembered that he would be home late that evening. For once I was thankful for the racketball game that would delay him.

I tried to persuade myself to settle down and stop being so upset. I might as well have been talking to kernels of popcorn in a pan of hot oil.

I pulled the bag of potatoes out of the pantry, and began peeling some. I worked so furiously, it was a wonder I had enough potatoes left to cook for dinner. Every time I came to a rotten spot on a potato, I thought to myself, *What a rotten mother you are. Your daughter is pregnant. Maybe. Oh, Lord, I don't think I can stand it. Please, don't let it be true.*

Once or twice, my mind touched on a picture of Sandy and Jim, sneaking off by themselves—I couldn't bear to think of it. After I'd trusted them both.

Somehow, the weekend passed. Sandy and I avoided each other. My husband asked me once if I didn't feel well; when I said I was fine, he hesitated a moment, but then said no more.

Monday came, finally, but not the phone call we waited for.

By Tuesday afternoon, not knowing was becoming unbearable. The only reason I could stand to wait was that I was desperately afraid that the worst might be true. At least, until I knew for sure, I had a little hope.

A few minutes before five o'clock that Tuesday, the call came. I recognized our physician's voice. "Sandy's test came back positive," he said. "If there is anything I can do to help, please let me know."

Slowly, I returned the receiver to its cradle. I stood there. On the desk in front of me lay a magazine, opened to a half-finished article. Next to it was a letter from my married daughter. On the wall hung a crewel picture I'd stitched. All those little details of life—none of them mattered now. I felt as if the woman who had opened that magazine, read that letter, stitched that picture, had simply disappeared. No, she was still there, but her world was gone.

With a start I realized that Sandy was standing in front of me. "Was that the doctor?"

I nodded.

"What did he say?"

I listened to myself reply. "The test came back positive."

Sandy turned abruptly and fled to her room.

I hadn't moved. I could still hear our physician's voice saying, "The test came back positive." No matter how hard he had tried to soften the blow, or how much concern had been reflected in his voice, his message was shattering.

I wanted to go to the kitchen and find something to eat, but my feet seemed stuck in cement. When my husband came through the front door a few minutes later, I was still standing next to the telephone.

He deposited the newspaper and his briefcase at the top of the stairs and turned to open the closet door. Then, as if he had suddenly realized that something was wrong, he stopped and stared at me. "What's the matter?" he asked.

When I didn't answer, he came and put his arms

around me. "What is it?" The tenderness in his voice triggered my tears. I tried to say, "Sandy is pregnant," but I couldn't do it. "Ask Sandy," I mumbled.

He turned and strode down the hall to her room. I heard her door open, and then I heard muffled voices. Tense, I waited; I knew he would be very angry and upset.

Before long, he came back. I was relieved, as well as surprised, that he was so calm. (What I didn't appreciate right then is that he simply had a different method for handling shock than I did. What showed on the surface didn't reflect at all what was inside.)

For a while, though, it was his apparent calm that we all leaned on. As for me, I couldn't shake the feeling that I had somehow been carried away from the world I knew and dumped unceremoniously in a strange land. Here, I knew neither who I was supposed to be, nor how I was supposed to behave.

Sleep that night, and for several that followed, seemed impossible. Over and over, my mind returned to the same questions. How am I ever going to get through this? Sandy's pregnant. Will life ever return to normal? Sandy's pregnant. . . .

Days passed. Neither Sandy nor I spoke much to each other. What was there to say?

I myself was trying to nurture a tiny seed of doubt, as illogical as that was. Maybe she isn't pregnant; the test could have been wrong. All the while, a still, small voice inside my head kept repeating, "You know she is. Why are you trying to fool yourself?"

In spite of hearing the diagnosis directly from our physician, and recognizing, finally, Sandy's very routine signs of early pregnancy, I still didn't want to believe it was true.

I longed for the days of maternal myopia, when motherly instincts had kept me from seeing that one of my children could possibly sin in such a manner.

After all, we had given her the best of Christian teaching and upbringing. Because our children had known biblical teachings about morality, I assumed they would never step beyond the established boundaries. How blind I'd been. I should have seen it coming.

For a while, I tried to cling to normality by doing what I normally would do. Except that I didn't normally forget what I had walked downstairs to get out of the freezer. Or leave the drapes closed all day, as if the sunshine mocked me. Or break out crying when a friend asked me if something was wrong.

Was something wrong? Was anything *right?*

I simply did not want to be the mother of an unwed mother. Why did I have to be involved, anyway? Didn't I have a choice?

Neither did I want anyone telling me, "God allows trials to come into our lives." All I wanted was an escape hatch.

Perhaps our pastor sensed that. We had called him to come that evening when we first knew for sure that Sandy was pregnant. Later, he must have realized how much I needed a sympathetic ear, because he simply showed up on my doorstep one day. He was wonderful. For almost an hour, without once glancing at his watch, he sat and let me talk.

It helped me a lot. Although he didn't try to give me any advice, I felt much better with my feelings out in the open. Now I saw what my first task had to be. I had to leap a formidable hurdle. I must accept the truth that Sandy was pregnant.

I wish I could say I leaped that hurdle as if I were a trapeze artist—flying through the air with the greatest of ease—but anyone who knows me would see through that in a minute. I made a lot of false starts, bruised my shins, and tried to get off the track altogether. Eventually, though, in spite of my own worst efforts, I made it.

2

From Reaction to Acceptance

"Just accept it. What else can you do, anyway?"

Both the unmarried pregnant girl and the person she turns to for help are bound to receive that advice sooner or later—if not from some other person, from themselves.

But saying to them, "Just accept it," is similar to telling one who is deeply depressed, "Just cheer up." It's not that the desire to do so is lacking. Desire alone isn't enough.

I remember how it was for me when I learned that Sandy was pregnant. I came to acceptance in a very roundabout way.

In the beginning, I simply denied that it could be true. I knew that if I kept busy enough, I wouldn't have time to think of it, so I cleaned the house from top to bottom, closets and all. That did wonders for appearances around home, but that's all. When I fell into bed at night, no matter how exhausted, the truth hovered over me, waiting to sneak through the slightest crevice in my resistance.

All right, then. If I had to think about it, I would, but only that. The knowledge might be in my mind, but I wouldn't let it into my heart, where it could do real damage.

But I didn't count on the clever spy system that sprang into action within me. It wasn't long until my carefully guarded head knowledge managed to infiltrate my inner being. No matter how hard I tried, I could not keep from feeling the pain in my heart. It was there. It hurt. I couldn't make it go away. Sandy was pregnant.

When crying didn't help and the pain seemed endless, I became angry. I'm not proud of myself, but I admit that I became so angry that I took it out on Sandy. She was, after all, the most obvious target.

For a while on that dismal Saturday afternoon, Sandy sat quietly—too quietly, it seemed to me. "How can you just sit there and act as if nothing is wrong?" I shouted at her.

"If I could change the truth, I would," she answered calmly. "But I can't. What do you want me to do, anyway?"

What did I want her to do? I wanted her not to be pregnant, that's what I wanted.

I didn't set out purposely to hurt her, but I couldn't seem to help myself. Not only did I not want to face the truth that she was pregnant, but I didn't want Sandy to have to face it either. I continued to pour out my frustrations on her.

Finally Sandy had enough. Tears began to gather in her eyes. She grabbed her purse, ran out the front door to her car, and drove off down the street.

"Go ahead, run off," I shouted after her. I was still angry, and becoming more so because now I felt I had to justify what I'd just said and done.

But why should I be sorry? I argued with myself. *Everything I said is true.* After a couple of hours, though, I found myself peeking through the living room curtains every time a car went by. Where was Sandy? What was she doing?

Supper time came, and I ate everything on my plate as well as anything else that was left on the table. I still had heard nothing from Sandy, and I began to worry in earnest.

What if she'd had an accident? What if she'd decided to run off somewhere? That's how a mother's mind seems to work. Why imagine less than the worst, if the worst might possibly happen?

The hours after supper stretched on and on. During those endless hours, I finally realized what the bottom line was. No matter what Sandy had done, I loved her and I wanted her to be home—with me, with her father, among people who truly cared about her.

Once again, at my normal, regrettably snail-like pace, I applied the advice I should have heeded much sooner: "Let all bitterness and wrath and anger and clamor and slander be put away from you, with all malice, and be kind to one another, tenderhearted, forgiving one another, as God in Christ forgave you" (Eph. 4:31, 32, RSV).

During those anxious hours, I discovered the key to my acceptance of Sandy's pregnancy. I had to stop thinking of myself, and to begin thinking of Sandy.

I had to face that deep chasm which separated my initial reaction from my ultimate acceptance, walk right up to the edge, and make the leap. The longer I hesitated, peering down at all those monsters—guilt, fear of the unknown, unwillingness to look truth in the eye, self-pity—the harder it would be to make myself jump.

It should have been easier, I think now. After all, I could call on my pastor or his wife any time I wanted to talk, and each of them is blessed with that rare talent of listening with the heart. Or on Christian friends, who were always ready to encourage and pray for me.

I knew, too, that God promises to supply the grace we need for any situation.

But before I could come to the point of acceptance, I

had to adjust my line of vision. I had to stop looking inward at me. Instead, I needed to focus on God as the source of love and wisdom, and indirectly on Sandy as one of God's children who was in need.

When Sandy finally appeared at the door that evening, I was waiting for her. "I'm sorry for what I said, honey," I told her. For the first time in a long time, I put my arms around my grown-up little girl and hugged her. "I don't know why it's been so much harder for me to accept the truth than it has been for you."

We went out in the kitchen, and I poured milk into a pan to heat.

As she stirred her hot chocolate, Sandy said, "It wasn't easier for me to get used to the idea; I just started working on it before you did."

It was past midnight before we turned out the kitchen light. Once we started sharing what was really going on inside us, it was hard to stop.

"I'm scared for you, Sandy, because I really don't know what lies ahead for you."

"I know; I am, too."

"You know I didn't mean to get so angry at you," I said.

Sandy shook her head. "Don't be sorry. Actually, while I was driving around this afternoon, I did a lot of thinking. And I decided that it was easier to have you angry at me than just ignoring me."

That surprised me. "What made you think I was ignoring you? I was just trying to keep myself calm."

Sandy took a deep breath. "I can see that now. But for a while, there, I thought you just didn't care about me at all."

Once we started, we found that we had a lot to talk about. When the sharing was over, I believe we both knew that a quiet transformation had occurred in our relationship. No longer would we be adult and little girl, or even just mother and daughter. Now we would also be woman and woman, friends.

Acceptance didn't come gracefully, or all at once, but come it did.

Others have found acceptance easier, and some have resisted as long as possible, or never found acceptance at all.

One woman I know told me that she and her husband guessed for several weeks that their unmarried daughter was pregnant. "I felt that I had accepted her pregnancy even before she had."

My sister related this incident. "I have a friend who had a terrible time accepting the truth that her unmarried daughter was pregnant. She traveled to several cities, trying to talk some relative, somewhere, into taking her daughter in until her baby was born."

Perhaps this unfortunate mother had assumed such a burden of guilt that the thought of looking upon her pregnant daughter, day in and day out, appeared unbearable.

"She told me she had thought she just couldn't accept it," my sister said. "But finally, she listened to her uncle, who convinced her that the best place for her daughter was at home."

For some, acceptance never comes. They may say to the pregnant girl, "You got yourself into this mess, now you can just get yourself out."

When my husband and I took Sandy to the hospital for her delivery, the nurse in charge told her, "You're a lucky girl to have someone to stand by you. We see many girls who have to come to the hospital in a taxi, or have a neighbor or friend drop them off. Nobody else could be bothered."

Her comment made me uneasy. I had been tempted to simply wash my hands of Sandy's pregnancy, so I'd better not sit in judgment of others who did the same thing.

What might I have done, I thought, without the

support I'd had from a faithful and loving God, from my pastor and his wife, and from praying friends and relatives?

Of course, although I had reached the point of acceptance, I did want to backtrack on occasion. I remember particularly how much I *didn't* want to go with Sandy when she shopped for maternity clothes. What if somebody I knew happened to see us?

Then, to the Spirit's gentle prodding, I agreed, "I know, your grace is sufficient." It was a truth I would come to understand to a far greater degree in the months ahead.

3

Don't Just Stand There; Tie Me Down
Or, how not to jump right in and stir up a hasty pudding.

All right. I accepted the reality of Sandy's pregnancy.
Then I sensed an urgency to move, and to move fast.
Plans must be planned, decisions decided, futures
foreseen. The sooner we all knew what Sandy was going
to do, the better off we'd all be.

That's what I thought. But I was wrong.

This pressure to spring into instant action proved to
stem from outdated attitudes that prevailed when I was
Sandy's age.

I think of the time when my husband and I set out
to show our children the apartment building in the city
where we had lived just after we were married.

Arriving at the intersection of Grant and 14th Street,
we were shocked. The building was gone. Not one
brick of it remained. A sea of cars, one of which stood
on the very spot where I prepared those first dinners,
inundated the parking lot.

However, if I had never gone back, I would still be
carrying in my mind a picture of that apartment building
as I knew it so many years ago—just as I now expected

to find attitudes toward the unwed mother the same as I had known then, too.

It doesn't seem so long ago that the girl who became pregnant before she married had (and expected to have) little to say about her future. For some, a quick wedding was arranged. Haste was the byword; indeed, a lack of haste demonstrated extremely poor taste. For others, it was a trip to a distant city "to visit an aunt." The object was not to show and never to tell, although the girl's flimsy excuse for leaving town seldom fooled anyone.

I was nine years old, or maybe ten, when one of my unmarried cousins became pregnant. It took me quite a long time to find out what all the flap was about. (We children knew that when the mothers were riled, the best thing we could do was to stay out of sight, or at least to keep quiet.)

I wondered what would happen next, but my aunt and my mother surely did not. No discussion was necessary. The course was clear; they would plan a wedding immediately.

If my cousin, the silly girl, wanted to sit upstairs and cry on her wedding day, that was her problem. "She should have thought of that sooner."

No one seemed at all concerned about the girl's ultimate good (or her baby's). The girl "had made her bed, and now she had to sleep in it."

No wonder I was surprised at the attitudes toward Sandy's pregnancy which I encountered time and again. They were completely different from those I'd grown up with.

If there is one word of encouragement I could pass on to anyone involved in an unwed pregnancy, it is this: it's not the same as it was. While the heartbreak hasn't changed, it seems that almost everything else has.

Maybe we've learned to become more honest in our appraisal of ourselves, and less likely to judge others. Or we've seen so many types of behavior via public media that we've become unshockable. Or we are better educated regarding the hidden factors behind the unwed pregnancy.

Whatever the reason, one thing is certain: the outlook for today's unwed mother is far more positive than it used to be.

Support replaces criticism. Calmness overrules panic. Once, the unwed pregnancy gave rise to hasty decisions, arrived at in an emotionally charged atmosphere and aggravated by an extreme sense of urgency. Uppermost in everyone's mind was how to cover up the girl's error.

Today the question is "How do we uncover what is best for this girl's personal potential?"

I first came across these unexpected attitudes at an agency in our city which provides a link between unmarried, pregnant girls and services available to them. I arrived anxious and left amazed. What had I expected? Maybe a certain subdued criticism or pious judgment or implied smugness. I couldn't have been more wrong.

To begin with, the woman who visited with Sandy and me was not at all what I'd thought she would be. Instead of a snooty-nosed, sour-faced old maid who would lecture us on our failures, I found an attractive, pleasant woman about my own age, who seemed concerned that we feel at ease.

"Hello. My name is Ruth," she said with a smile. "Please come in and have a seat." She explained that she was a volunteer, and that she came to the office once a week, but would be happy to visit at other times with Sandy or me if that would help.

Within minutes, I began to catch a faint glimmer of hope that I could relax and stop waiting for the hatchet to fall. I had another surprise coming, too.

When Ruth asked Sandy what she had thought of doing, I immediately spoke up. "Well, the first thing Sandy needs to do is to get busy and decide just that."

Once more, to my increasing perplexity, I was wrong. Gracefully but firmly, Ruth impressed upon me that I was in error.

"Most people feel that way," she said. "It does appear as if that would be good. But actually," she said with a smile toward Sandy, "the girl often doesn't know what she wants to do for quite a while. It's better not to rush her."

I made up my mind to keep quiet for the rest of the visit.

Ruth then opened a large reference book and began to go through it with Sandy. First she turned to a section about social service agencies. "This agency maintains a home where girls can stay if they can't live at home," Ruth explained. "And this one is run by the Catholic Church. This one handles only adoptions. Here is one that assists girls who may wish to be single parents."

She turned to another section. "This lawyer will provide legal services at a reduced rate, if you need his help," Ruth said. And later, "Do you need financial assistance?"

For the next half hour, Ruth pointed out to Sandy all the different avenues of service that were open to her. As they visited, I waited for Ruth to exhibit any sign of criticism, any negative attitude at all.

It never came. When we left, I felt as if someone had handed me a one-hundred-dollar bill, and I still couldn't believe it was genuine.

Probably Ruth is just unusual, I decided. Attitudes couldn't have changed that much.

Over and over again, though, I found that they had. Wherever Sandy went—to the physician's office, to work, to church—she was greeted matter-of-factly as a pregnant woman. If anyone felt called upon to express criticism, he or she certainly did not do so openly.

What a difference this can make. If only every unwed mother understood this.

Some young girls are so afraid of revealing their pregnancy that they nearly starve themselves in an effort to hide their condition for as long as they can. This is most unfortunate, as this practice can cause serious damage to their unborn babies.

Because of unfounded fears, an unwed mother may resort to other desperate measures to keep her secret.

Recently, a young single girl in our city became pregnant and then hid away in an apartment during her entire pregnancy. All alone, she gave birth to a baby girl. Two days later, this infant was found in a trash can in a city park; a passing jogger had heard the infant's crying.

This baby girl lived. But my heart cried out for her and her mother. If only this unwed mother had known what help and support could have been hers, had she only asked. She need not have hidden away, lonely and miserable, during her pregnancy, nor endured the trauma of labor and delivery, frightened and alone. Nor need she have been so desperate that she tried to dispose of her baby in a trash can.

That certainly isn't necessary in today's world. Regardless of the choice an unmarried pregnant girl ultimately makes for her future, she can expect to find social, legal, and spiritual support.

I wish I had realized sooner the difference in attitudes which Sandy would encounter. The pressure I felt to get busy and do something only led to unnecessary frustration for all of us.

For instance, I rushed off to a lawyer and demanded that he put the wheels in motion immediately to bring about justice in Sandy's situation. That was a mistake. Later I would see that the wheels of justice turn rather slowly and nothing could be done finally until the baby was born.

(However, for possible legal purposes, the pregnant girl should save any items that may prove pertinent: letters or other written statements in which the baby's father states his intention to marry her; pictures, jewelry, or other gifts; and all receipts for expenses related to her pregnancy.)

I nagged at Sandy to hurry up and decide what she would do with the rest of her life, as if the only reason she hadn't already done so was that she wasn't trying hard enough.

Meanwhile, the days and weeks were passing; it wouldn't be long before Sandy's secret became public knowledge. Pregnancy can be *so* obvious. Even though I couldn't think what to do, I still felt as if I had to hurry.

I wish someone had taken me by the scruff of the neck and said, "Stop it. You aren't getting anywhere with all this wasted motion."

In a way, that is what the Lord did. I was reading in 1 Thessalonians, chapter five, and I stopped when I came to verse 18. ". . . give thanks in all circumstances; for this is the will of God in Christ Jesus for you" (RSV). Could it be possible that *I* was supposed to give thanks in *my* circumstances? I protested. "Lord, look at what is happening in my life. How can you tell me to give thanks?"

Once I began to give thanks, regardless of my circumstances, I found it made sense to do so. I could not possibly be running in two directions at once. If I was busy giving thanks, I couldn't be worrying. If my mind was stayed on God, I couldn't be downcast over my present state of affairs.

About this time, I began to understand more perfectly what Paul meant when he said that "tribulation worketh patience." If I would be patient, God would work out his will for Sandy.

And really, very little needs to be decided upon immediately. But the pregnant girl does need to make the decision, as soon as she can, to love her baby.

4

Love the Baby

Or, I'm depending on you, Mom.

Most of the questions which worry the pregnant girl do not need an immediate answer. But one question does: will she love her baby?

But why would I say that? All mothers love their babies.

But do they? If so, then why are so many babies being destroyed before they even draw their first breath?

Consider the unwed pregnancy from the girl's point of view. This new life within her may represent only heartache, indecision, and frustration. In addition, any woman pregnant with her first child can experience a legitimate concern about her capability to be a truly good mother.

The pregnant girl can get so caught up in the negative aspects of her pregnancy that she fails to recognize the miracle of conception that has occurred.

Hers isn't an illegitimate baby; it is a baby whose parents failed to legitimize their relationship. In the sight of God, this baby has the same rights as any other baby.

The woman who does not acknowledge these rights, but who chooses abortion instead, turns her back on God's promise to work all things together for good. Christ himself has dignified our humanity by assuming it. We ought not, then, to dishonor the humanity in even the very humblest.

Who could be more humble than an unborn baby, who is entirely at the mercy of his mother? If the mother says, "This is my body, and I want to control it; I don't want any baby getting in my way," the baby is helpless and vulnerable.

Actually, I see nothing wrong with a woman's wishing to control her body. But I do see everything wrong when she fails to exercise control at the proper time, and then forces an innocent child to pay for her mistake.

According to a recent survey, thirty of every one hundred babies conceived in the United States are aborted. Adolescent mothers, who represent only 18 percent of all women of child-bearing age, had 31 percent of the abortions.

Abortion may have moved from the ghetto of secret shame to the glitter of the political arena. But political rhetoric cannot make it right. Psalm 22:10 says, "I was cast upon thee from the womb: thou art my God from my mother's belly" (KJV).

God knows each baby as soon as it is conceived. At the moment of conception, as soon as the twenty-three chromosomes contained in both the sperm and the egg meet, that one cell has complete within it the forty-six chromosomes which make up the entire genetic code of a human being.

Still, when a poll of registered voters in 1980 indicated that 78 percent of them favored allowing abortion, presidential candidates found it necessary to address the issue of abortion. Of course, politicians don't go looking for controversial issues on which to take a stand. Often, though, they are pressured into doing so by organizations such as NOW (the National Organization for Women).

NOW includes in its Bill of Rights " . . . the right of women to control their own reproductive lives by . . . access to contraceptive information and devices, and by repealing penal laws governing abortion."

The American Civil Liberties Union has published the following statement in *The Rights of Americans:*

There can be no justification for statutory categories that seek to limit the lawfulness of abortions by the physical or mental circumstances of the mother or fetus; lawful abortions should instead be freely available to every woman at her option.

I strongly disagree. And yet I sense that abortion has come to be acceptable to many people.

Francis Schaeffer and C. Everett Koop, M.D., address this problem in their book, *Whatever Happened to the Human Race?*

They explain how what was morally "unthinkable" only years ago is "thinkable" now. Even some among the medical profession, the authors point out, have recognized a new thinkable. Some institutions have deleted the phrase, "from the time of conception," from the Hippocratic Oath clause beginning, "I will maintain the utmost respect for human life."

I wondered, too, how many women who have an abortion are anxious to let it be known? I believe that those actions we take, all the while hoping that no one will find out about them, are usually wrong.

Regardless of how sure a woman may feel that she desires an abortion, how will she feel later on in her life? Will she think well of herself?

Once pregnant, a woman's body begins to make biological and emotional preparation for motherhood.

What happens if her pregnancy is prematurely terminated? Koop and Schaeffer relate the following reaction.

One woman, as she suffered the aftereffects of a recommended abortion, asked:

"Why didn't anyone tell me I would feel like a mother with empty arms? Why didn't anyone tell me I risked spoiling the possibility of having a normal pregnancy, because of the damage that might be done to my body by the abortion?"

. . . Abortion counselors rarely talk about physical dangers, emotional results and psychological consequences. They seldom tell the woman what is going to happen or what may be involved.

In the light of all of the publicity about abortion, it is highly likely that the possibility of choosing this "solution" may occur to the pregnant girl, or to the person who wants to help her.

Although it is hard for me to admit, during one particularly bleak period of time, I did allow the possibility of abortion to linger in my mind. To be more precise, I dwelt on the thought of how much better off both Sandy and I would be if she were not pregnant, while I tried to stifle the thought of the dead baby. It didn't work.

Later, I prayed that God would forgive me for even thinking of abortion. I know well that God views each life as unique and precious, that life depends on him. "He is before all things, and in him all things hold together" (Col. 1:17, RSV).

A friend of mine who became pregnant almost ten years after her youngest child was born, told me, "The first thing the nurse asked me when she came back into the room was, 'Do you want an abortion?' I was shocked, but she said she always asks that question nowadays."

Another friend called a local obstetrician's office to

make an appointment to confirm her pregnancy. The receptionist asked her over the telephone if she was considering an abortion. She chose another physician.

However, this is the atmosphere in which today's woman lives. Pregnancy, even in marriage, is often regarded as a cause for sympathy, rather than for rejoicing.

The advice, "Abortion is all right; it's what you want that counts," bombards our young women today. Often, this advice penetrates and becomes a part of a woman's thinking even though she does not consciously acknowledge or accept it.

This is why I would say to the unwed mother, "Decide to love your baby." This is a vital decision, one that needs to be made as quickly as possible.

Armed with this decision, this act of her will to choose to love her baby, the pregnant girl can defend herself against the temptation to abort her baby. The battle can be over before it begins; she won't allow any harm to come to a baby she loves.

Other people close to the pregnant girl can help in this matter, too. They can create an atmosphere which encourages love for her baby. One way to do this is to speak with respect and reverence toward the new life her baby represents. The kind and loving tone of voice she hears from other people can inspire a like response from the pregnant girl.

Most important, the Holy Spirit is available to help instill in the pregnant girl's heart a deep love for her baby. As the Spirit works, the pregnant girl can know beyond a doubt that she does love her child, and that she wants to do all she can to protect and nurture that child.

In Sandy's case, her immediate and firm stance was against abortion. I was thankful for that. For her, the decision to love her baby also meant that she took proper care of herself and that she thought ahead to the future in terms of what was best for her baby.

At last, here was a positive step I could take to help. I called the obstetrician who had deliverd my youngest child and set up an appointment for Sandy.

I didn't look forward to walking in to his office with an unmarried, pregnant daughter, since the people there all knew me. But that didn't matter nearly as much as knowing that Sandy (and her baby) would be receiving the best of care.

How important is adequate prenatal supervision? According to research done by the March of Dimes, an organization dedicated to protecting against birth defects, the answer is: *very important.*

The baby of a pregnant woman may be in danger *if:*

She doesn't see a doctor right away. The obstetrician or physician is the only one qualified to manage a pregnancy. He can detect potential problems in their early stages when preventive measures can be effective. And he can give advice concerning the best program of nutrition, rest, and exercise for each individual patient.

This is especially important for the very young mother. According to public health statistics, infants of very young mothers (particularly those under the age of fifteen) are more likely to be born prematurely, underweight, or incapable of surviving.

She doesn't eat enough of the right foods. For many of today's young people, a balanced meal is one that doesn't tip on the fast-food tray. Although her physician may prescribe supplemental vitamins and minerals, it is still imperative that the pregnant woman consume enough of the proper nutrients every day.

Her physician will also monitor her weight gain. While he won't want to see a gain that is extemely above the norm, he may not be as strict as he might have been a few years ago. Excessive weight gain can make delivery and recovery more difficult. Still, the physician does not want the baby to get inadequate nutrients because the mother is eating too little, or too little of the right foods.

Often a physician will provide handbooks which include information on the pregnant woman's diet. Or, information about nutrition (and other useful materials) can be obtained from the Consumer Information Center, Pueblo, Colorado 81009. Simply write and ask them for a copy of their Consumer Information Catalog, which lists materials available and tells how to order them.

She drinks. (No one knows how much is too much.) Drinking beer, wine, or liquor can lead to fetal alcohol syndrome and might contribute to growth problems, hyperactivity, retardation, heart defects, and other birth defects.

In addition, the Food and Drug Administration has recently issued a warning to pregnant women regarding the use of products that contain caffeine: coffee, tea, cola drinks, chocolate, and some medications. Final evidence of their harmful effect is not yet in, but the FDA does advise expectant mothers either to abstain from or to practice moderation in the use of products containing caffeine.

She smokes. In a report by former Surgeon General Dr. Julius B. Richmond, he warns that an expectant mother who smokes is likely to deliver a lower-weight baby who may suffer behavioral problems or stunted intellectual development. Also, she risks increased incidence of spontaneous abortion (miscarriage), fetal death, death of a newborn baby, or sudden infant death syndrome.

She takes drugs. According to Dr. Conway Hunter, who is associated with an addictive disease treatment unit at an Atlanta, Georgia, hospital, "The toxic effect of one joint of marijuana cigarette is equal to five packs of cigarettes in its damage to the lungs.

"It is very damaging to the brain, primarily. . . . It damages the reproductive system, causes impotence, chromosomal changes and fetal abnormalities."

Marijuana has an affinity for the brain and the sex organs.

Dr. Akira Morishima, of Columbia University, further points out, "A human female is born with about 400,000 eggs. If they are injured, there's no way to repair that damage. It has been proven that . . . the mind-altering substances in marijuana accumulate in the ovaries, as well as in other organs."

And this is "only" marijuana. Babies of mothers who are addicted to stronger drugs often must endure withdrawal symptoms after their birth, and may suffer permanent damage.

She has veneral disease.
She is under eighteen.
Birth defects run in either family.
Any of these three circumstances will serve as a warning sign to her physician. If he knows of them early enough, the physician may be able to begin treatment according-ly and prevent unneccessary or avoidable defects in the infant.

One of the best ways to supplement the information an obstetrician or physician provides is by attending a prenatal class he recommends.

When Sandy told me that she had been advised to sign up for a prenatal class, my first reaction was, "Great." But when she asked if I would go with her, I was less enthusiastic.

Both of us knew she should go. But we were also apprehensive about how we would be treated.

As it turned out, our fears were totally unfounded.

When we arrived for the first of four classes, which were conducted at the hospital where Sandy would deliver her baby, we slipped in at the last minute and took seats at the back of the room.

As I surveyed the room, I noticed that the majority of people there were couples, but also there were several women by themselves, or with another woman.

As the nurse in charge spoke, I began to relax. "The main reason I'm here tonight is selfish," she said. "The more the pregnant woman knows about what to expect and how to help in her delivery, the easier my job is. And the better she takes care of herself while she is pregnant, the easier she can expect her delivery to be."

I became aware, as she talked, that she was always careful to refer to the baby's mother and father as "you and your partner," not "you and your husband."

Her attitude seemed to be, "I care about helping you to have the best pregnancy and delivery possible, not about how you happened to become pregnant."

As I sat through those classes, I couldn't help but wish that I'd had an opportunity to attend such a class before my first baby was born. Whoever said ignorance is bliss had to be someone who never gave birth to a baby.

The first class dealt with the mother's nutritional needs, and what she should be doing about rest and activity levels.

A film was shown at the second class; it detailed the development of the unborn baby from conception to birth (including a picture of an unborn baby sucking his thumb).

At the third session, the nurse began to emphasize preparation for labor and delivery. She explained all of the different stages of labor and the terms that the personnel would be using. Then she demonstrated breathing techniques to be used during labor. "Did you know that a lack of oxygen increases pain?" she asked, whereupon class participation picked up remarkably. I even found myself going "pant-pant-breathe."

The class was then taken on a tour of the maternity wing. The nurse pointed out a fetal monitor and also the viewing screens in the nurses' station on which data from the fetal monitors was observed. The tour then proceeded to the delivery room, where she explained what the equipment was all about. (I was amazed at how different a delivery room looked when I was standing up.)

At the fourth and final session, postpartum care of the mother and care of the newborn baby were covered. A packet of free sample materials from several manufacturers of baby products was distributed to each mother-to-be.

Throughout all of the sessions, the emphasis was always on providing quality care for the pregnant woman and her baby.

If a pregnant girl is reluctant to attend prenatal classes, I think she should be encouraged to go anyway. As I said, nobody made Sandy feel out of place. I am sure that most pregnant girls, even if unmarried, would find the same sort of acceptance.

The important thing, though, is that she will be thankful for the knowledge she gained earlier when it is time for her labor and delivery.

Long before this momentous time arrives, however, the pregnant girl needs to do some of the most serious thinking she may ever do in all of her life. She needs to begin considering what her options are for her own and her baby's future.

I could help Sandy care for her physical needs. But I felt helpless when it came to helping her think through what was best for the future. It wasn't that I didn't want to help her; I was simply too emotionally involved.

For that reason, I encouraged Sandy to begin visiting a qualified Christian counselor.

5

The Christian Counselor
*Or, two heads are better than one,
when one of them isn't mine.*

When Sandy became pregnant, she had no choice but to make a giant step from adolescence to the best form of maturity she could muster. My role in her life had to change accordingly, too.

All of this change had to be accomplished at the worst possible time, a time when our emotional muscles were already stretched to the limit of their endurance. How would we adjust?

For both of us, the needed help came from Christian counselors who observed us and pointed out flaws in our performance. They helped us open our minds to new ideas, to direct our energies toward positive goals.

We learned the value of Ephesians 4:23: "And be renewed in the spirit of your minds" (RSV).

At first, Sandy resisted the idea of counseling. She admitted she was confused, but she was afraid a counselor would tell her what she must do. Although she was unsure what plans she wanted to make, she did want to make them herself.

When I tried to explain how hard that could be, she said, "Then you help me decide."

But I couldn't. I simply could not be sure what I was putting first—her best interests or mine. I sensed that it would be impossible to be both normal and neutral.

Too much hinged on the answers she chose for so many important questions. For instance, what would she do when her baby was born? I didn't believe Sandy was ready to accept the responsibility for raising a child. I knew I didn't want to do it for her. And that left adoption; I couldn't imagine how any woman could choose that, either.

This was just one of many difficult questions Sandy faced. I was only beginning to realize that Sandy would encounter pain no matter how carefully she answered these questions. Many of her choices offered only painful solutions; I didn't want to be the one who had advised her which choice to make.

When Sandy finally agreed to visit a counselor, it was a great relief to me. And it was to Sandy, too, once she found she wouldn't be pushed into a decision she didn't want to make.

"I still am not sure what I want to do," Sandy told me after her second visit with her counselor, "but I'm beginning to see why I'm having such a big struggle."

One benefit Sandy received from counseling was a widening of her perspective. She needed to stop thinking only of her present circumstances, and to begin to consider what she could still accomplish in all her years ahead.

She showed me a verse in her *Living Bible* which her counselor had pointed out to her: "So we do not look at what we can see right now, the troubles all around us, but we look forward to the joys in heaven which we have not yet seen. The troubles will soon be over, but the joys to come will last forever" (2 Cor. 4:18).

"You know," Sandy said, "I felt that my life was over, or that it might as well be. I felt as if I had ruined my chances forever for a good life."

It surprised Sandy when her counselor wanted to administer some tests to discover what her capabilities were. She was so caught up in misery over her present predicament that she had stopped thinking beyond it. It encouraged her very much to talk about how to go on with her education, and how she could live to her fullest potential.

Perhaps one of the greatest helps Sandy received was learning how to find release from the shame and guilt she felt. Her counselor pointed out to her Psalm 103: 10-14: "He does not deal with us according to our sins, nor requite us according to our iniquities. For as the heavens are high above the earth, so great is his steadfast love toward those who fear him; as far as the east is from the west, so far does he remove our transgressions from us. As a father pities his children, so the Lord pities those who fear him. For he knows our frame; he remembers that we are dust" (RSV).

Sandy's counselor pointed out that God has forgiven others for the sin of premarital sex, and he would also forgive her.

Because I recognized that God doesn't go around administering doses of forgiveness here and there the way mothers used to give out spring tonic—just in case of need—I prayed often that Sandy would repent of and ask forgiveness for her sin. I myself knew the peace which follows forgiveness, and I desired that same peace for her, too.

Sometimes, in all our efforts to convey to the unwed mother our understanding and sympathy, we may fail ever to say to her, "But yet, you must tell God you're sorry for what you did." All of the counseling in the world isn't going to replace the forgiveness of God when it comes to restoring peace within her soul.

Equally important, though, is that once she has asked for and received forgiveness, the pregnant girl need not go on thinking of herself as a second-class Christian. A girl who has borne a child out of wedlock may even wonder if she has the right to marry. I believe that a girl who has received God's forgiveness for this sin is as good as new in his sight; therefore, she has every right to marry.

One important result of counseling is that the pregnant girl can gain proper insights, thereby regaining her self-esteem and returning to a life of useful service to God.

She needs to understand the reason for her behavior. If she does not, she may very well fall victim to circumstances again.

Often, girls are driven by motivations they don't understand. In his booklet, *Counseling with the Unwed Mother*, Dr. Clyde M. Narramore points out the following motivations:

—*Lack of acceptance from her parents: she seeks affection through the illicit love affair.*
—*Inadequate teaching of moral codes and standards.*
—*Lack of commitment to God: power to control the sex drive is strengthened by a dedicated life in Christ.*
—*The desire to be accepted by peers: she needs the approval of others, so chooses to follow the crowd.*
—*Lack of sex education: the girl learns through experience, rather than through teaching.*
—*The victim of the exploiter: she may innocently fall for a man whose only intention is to use her physically.*
—*To punish her parents: because she has strong feelings of rejection, her pregnancy is an attempt to hurt her parents.*
—*Desire to get married: if her parents object to her marriage, she may feel that a pregnancy will end their objections.*
—*To hold on to a fading relationship: she sees the*

pregnancy as a lever to force her boyfriend to marry her.
—*Lack of definite aims or worthwhile life plans: she drifts into premarital sex relations because she has no meaningful goals in her life.*

I believe that for her to know what happens *if* she yields isn't as important as for her to know *why* she yields.

A good counselor can help her to understand why she behaved as she did. With this knowledge, the girl can insulate herself against future temptation. " . . . Make straight paths for your feet, so that what is lame may not be put out of joint but rather be healed" (Heb. 12:13, RSV).

While Sandy was receiving counsel, I needed some, too. How did I rid myself of a nagging feeling of guilt? Did I have the right to limit the changes I would tolerate in my life style? Why was it necessary for me to be forthright and honest with Sandy about my feelings?

Guilt can be common to anyone, parent or friend, who is close to an unwed mother. Although we are not responsible, we assume a sense of guilt.

I remember my thoughts. Maybe I should have been stricter. What if we had waited a year before we moved, until Sandy finished her last year in high school? I probably should have explained the facts of life better than I did. Why didn't I stop her from seeing so much of him?

In other words, if I had done something differently, this might not have happened. So, in a way, it was my fault, too.

Oh? Was it? Assumed guilt is really nothing more than a device the devil uses to keep our thoughts turned inward. The longer we allow guilt to linger, the longer we are saying, "Look at me; look at what I did."

The Bible says that "no temptation has overtaken you that is not common to man . . ." (1 Cor. 10:13, RSV). And to our children, then, too. Although I don't mean to imply that this in any way justifies Sandy's actions, it would have helped me to maintain a better outlook if I had borne this in mind.

I needed to stop and think. Is yielding to the temptation to indulge in premarital intercourse a greater sin than yielding to the temptation to, say, spread gossip? Or is the result of the first only more obvious?

Actually, I knew on one level that I shouldn't feel guilty. But it was only through counseling that I could act on what I knew and lay aside this guilt.

I had to acknowledge that the ultimate responsibility for Sandy's pregnancy was not mine, but hers. I had to say that I had done the best I could to raise her with the right values. I needed to feel responsive to Sandy's needs, but not responsible for her choices.

It's easy to second-guess myself at this point. For instance, I wish I'd never said, concerning some issue of discipline, "Oh, just this once, it won't matter." What kind of example did that provide for Sandy when she was battling temptation?

But I *didn't* know then what I know now. I *did* do the best I could with the knowledge I then had.

My counselor also encouraged me to be open with Sandy. "You have a right to tell your daughter exactly how you feel about your hopes for your own future," she said.

That caused a problem for me. Here I was, with grown children, plus our youngest who was about to enter school. I was looking forward to some free time again, not to having another baby around the house.

Yet, when I thought of explaining this to Sandy, I felt as if I were being selfish.

It caused tension between my husband and me, too. He loves babies—as long as someone else is taking care of them—and he wanted Sandy to bring up her baby in our home.

But I see too often what that means to Grandmother. She becomes a surrogate mother. After all, what is she going to do when her daughter goes back to school or to work, let some stranger take care of her little darling?

Before I had any grandchildren, I suspected that a lot of this grandparent business was nothing more than a big put-on. I guess a person has to be a grandparent before he or she can understand how each grandchild can be the most precious child in the world.

Still, I had plans and goals for my life that didn't include a new baby in the household. What should I do? More than that, what did I have the right to do?

My counselor listened carefully, and when I asked her these questions, she answered very directly. "You have several rights in this situation," she said. "You certainly have the right to tell your daughter exactly what you are willing to do for her."

In other words, if Sandy were to get married, would I allow her and her husband and baby to live in our home? Would I provide child care—and, if so, how often and how long—if she didn't marry but kept her baby? If she continued to live at home, was I willing to go on indefinitely washing her clothes and putting away her curling iron?

"Stake out your boundaries," my counselor advised. "Establish what your limits are. Otherwise, you are going to feel boxed in and trapped by circumstances. This can only lead to frustration and friction in your home."

I should tell Sandy exactly what she could expect from me. "In that way, Sandy can base her decisions on facts, not on assumptions which could prove to be false."

Moreover, I had to be honest with myself. I would love to be a grandmother, but not a mother again.

It wasn't easy, but I did speak with Sandy. "I am

willing to allow you and your baby to stay here for six months. After that time, I will want you to establish your own home. When it fits into my schedule, I will be happy to baby-sit for you, but I won't necessarily be available any time you ask."

As I look at these words on the page, they appear to be unkind. But I believe I would have been far less kind if I had not been open and direct with Sandy. At least, as she considered her and her baby's futures, she knew exactly what she could expect from me. I didn't let her make plans that assumed more (or less) assistance from me than I was ready to give.

Because the counselor can play such an important role in our lives, it is important to select the right one.

The professional counselor who is also a Christian is the ideal choice for a believer seeking help. This counselor will be best qualified to perceive whether our need is in the physical, emotional, or spiritual realm.

While he recognizes the value of prayer, he won't insist that more diligent prayer is the only answer for emotional stress, any more than he would recommend aspirin if we had difficulty praying.

How do you locate this person? Usually, once he or she establishes a practice, the churches in the surrounding area become familiar with his or her name. You may know of someone who has received good counseling, and ask that person for a referral. Or you could check with the mental health unit of a hospital or with a mental health clinic in your area.

Another choice for counsel is your minister or pastor. However, if you feel constrained to be on your best behavior around him and can't admit that you'd like to kick the dog when nobody is looking, then your minister may not be your best choice. The counselor's task of helping us to discern our true feelings is hard enough when we are being completely open. When we are actively concealing portions of ourselves, his task is thwarted before he begins.

Occasionally a lay person is blessed of God with ability to counsel. I received my counseling from a woman who has informal training, but who possesses an innate ability to help the individual who is hurting.

Take care, though, when choosing the lay counselor. The best of intentions do not necessarily make a good counselor.

Indeed, scratch beneath the surface of many people, and you will uncover an amateur advisor. For these people, the urge to pass on advice is almost irresistible. Perhaps the best criterion for judging whether or not to accept such advice is whether or not you requested it.

On the other hand, many people shared our concern, and did so by telling of some experience that had happened to them or to someone close to them. In some cases, they divulged secrets that had been hidden for years. I appreciated their desire to show kindness. In effect, each one said, "I know what you're going through. I've been there myself."

Occasionally, though, I sensed that Sandy was confused by conflicting points of view. "When that happens," I told her, "thank that person for sharing with you and ask them to pray that you will know God's will for your life."

It would be good if everyone could remember that the unwed mother's mind may already be in turmoil. For her to receive a wide variety of opinions and advice only increases her uncertainty.

For her own well-being, she needs to zero in on the one counselor she has chosen. This person is in the best position to help uncover the course of action that is most fitted to the individual girl's potential.

A counselor can accomplish much that a parent or friend can not. But he can't take our place.

The friend or parent has two big advantages: we are easier to see, and our time comes free.

During Sandy's pregnancy, she and I came to know each other very well. Through sharing her difficulty, the bond of love between us grew.

Many times Sandy simply needed company. She was different from her friends, and didn't get included in their plans. Even when she did see them, she discovered they weren't very grown-up.

So she and I spent lots of time together. We played countless games of Scrabble; we sewed; we shopped; we picked apples and canned pickles together.

I learned to cultivate ways of showing affection, too. For Sandy, a hug or squeeze of the hand was like rain on parched ground.

While the counselor is helpful, he or she cannot take the place of the loyal friend. On the other hand, he can help to make "our place" more peaceful during this troubled time.

One area in particular may have caused us far greater stress without the insight Sandy and I received in counseling. Should Sandy get married?

Marry, Marry, Quite Contrary

Must the single pregnant girl marry? Should she?
Is it possible to disagree peacefully?

Probably the very next question the single pregnant girl is asked after "Are you sure?" is "Are you going to get married?"

Old habits are hard to break, even when their track record proves to be very poor. I can understand why a person would want to believe that marriage at this point will solve all problems. However, to continue to believe so in the face of proven failure is not so easy to understand.

Some churches encourage premarital guidelines, which include a six-month wait between engagement and wedding, even in the case of pregnancy.

This is a response to statistics indicating that one in four marriages ends in divorce; that 50 percent of marriages involving teenagers fail; and that *90 percent* of teenage marriages prompted by pregnancy fail.

I had my own reasons for hoping that Sandy would not marry Jim. First, Jim was not a believer. Second, I sensed that Sandy was unsure that the marriage would succeed.

The question was how to approach her without causing hard feelings. As our pastor has said, "It's not our differences that cause problems; it's how we handle our differences."

I prayed that the Lord would help me to handle this difference in a way that would result in a peaceful resolution, and one that was acceptable to him.

A friend, sharing in Sunday school, provided me with the answer I needed. From her *Living Bible*, she read Psalm 94:19: "Lord, when doubts fill my mind, when my heart is in turmoil, quiet me and give me renewed hope and cheer."

How often my heart was in turmoil those days. It's not easy to watch a young couple break up. And it becomes less easy to watch when the girl is pregnant, especially if she can't seem to accept that all that was good in their relationship is over, no matter how much she may wish otherwise.

On several occasions, I was tempted to step in and say to Sandy, "Just forget Jim; you're better off without him, anyway." Then I would remember: "Quiet me. . . ." Instead of talking to Sandy, I talked to God. "Help her to know your will and help me to keep quiet."

It wasn't as long as it seemed before Sandy came to me and said, "I've decided not to marry Jim."

I could see that she was trying not to cry. I reached out and took her in my arms and hugged her. How thankful I was for that "quiet me."

"And Mom," she said, "thanks for not telling me what to do." Oops, now two of us needed handkerchiefs.

Sandy and I reached another turning point that day. Once she realized that I wasn't going to push my wishes on her, she felt free to talk over with me whatever was on her mind. Even though we didn't always think *alike*, at least we could think *together*.

The pregnant girl who is struggling over the decision

to marry or not to marry might benefit from sitting down with a trusted friend and considering the following thoughts.

She does not have to get married. I touched on this before, but I feel it is important to emphasize it. Too many people still do not realize how much attitudes toward the unwed mother have changed.

A couple of weeks ago, my friends' daughter Kim, who is sixteen, told me how her girl friend became eighteen, pregnant, and married—in that order.

"I feel so sorry for her," Kim said. "Her boyfriend was already mean to her before they were married, and I know she didn't really want to go through with the wedding."

When I asked Kim why her girl friend did go ahead, then, Kim looked at me with surprise written all over her face. "Well, they had to," she said.

Inwardly, I sighed. Notions like these take such hold on us that we never question them. It wasn't so long ago since I too would have said, "They had to."

It just is not true. Today's unwed mother *does not* have to get married. She might even choose to postpone marriage until after her baby is born.

With the proper support, she can find her pregnancy far less unbearable than she had expected.

Has she faced the question of her partner's relationship to God? Recently, a friend told me how her daughter almost broke off her engagement. Her fiance was not willing to participate in devotions with her before their marriage.

"She felt that it was his place to lead them in spiritual matters, and she told him she wouldn't marry him unless he was willing to begin that leading right away."

It is wonderful to hear of a young person with such strong convictions.

If the pregnant girl's partner is not a Christian, she needs to honor her convictions, too. Knowing the command in 2 Corinthians 6:14 (RSV): "Do not be mismated with unbelievers. . . ." isn't enough. She needs to abide by this command.

In her present state of mind (not to mention physical condition), the pregnant girl may believe you are being most unkind if you make an issue of this matter. How can you even suggest that she not marry him?

Perhaps she has confused kindness with weakness. What may appear to be the kind action at the moment—allowing her to go ahead and marry an unbeliever—may prove to be just the opposite not too far down the road. If her wishes are weakly accepted at this point in the mistaken belief that it is the kind thing to do, she may learn too late that she was wrong.

However, once we have spoken directly to her, we need to turn the entire matter over to God. As I need to be reminded often, God can accomplish much more if I get out of his way.

When I talked with Sandy about marriage, I emphasized that God sets down rules which are designed to improve our quality of living, not to interfere with our happiness. The rule against the marriage of a believer to an unbeliever is a prime example of his wisdom.

If her young man agrees to marriage, but expresses some reluctance, what then? Above all, the pregnant girl needs to be certain that he is not marrying her simply because he feels a duty to do so. This can result in his feeling trapped by the marriage. He may attempt to relieve the resulting frustration he experiences by venting it on what he perceives to be its source—his wife.

On the other hand, if the young man is given

enough time, and feels free to make his own choice, he may decide that marriage is what he wants.

If he is secretly against marriage, however, the pregnant girl is far better off knowing his true feelings before any vows are spoken. Although she may find it hard to believe at the moment, her decision not to marry under these circumstances is probably one she will be glad for later on.

What happens to the girl who wants very much to get married, but whose partner does not? She will experience painful feelings of rejection, but she need not be utterly devastated. She can be helped in at least two ways.

First, by understanding what his reasons may have been for refusing to marry her.

Perhaps he just isn't ready to get married—not to her, not to anyone. What is his background? If his parents' marriage is poor, he may wish to avoid a similar situation.

If he is quite young, he may not be able to accept the responsibility of a wife and child (and this may be true even if he is not so young). Some people have an unreasonable fear of responsibility regardless of their age.

He may not be able to love anyone but himself.

In essence, then, it may help the pregnant girl if she realizes that her young man's rejection of marriage isn't necessarily a rejection of her.

Second, we can make our loving support freely evident. Experiencing rejection, whether real or apparent, is painful. Our love and concern can hasten her recovery and alleviate some of her pain.

How can she be helped to release the partner who does not wish to marry her? Perhaps the only way to approach the girl who is clinging desperately to a very reluctant partner is to appeal to her love for him.

What does she believe would make him happier? Buying mag wheels for his car, or a washing machine to launder diapers? Would he rather run a household, or just run around?

True love isn't selfish. It puts the needs and desires of the other person first. Is she thinking first of him, or of herself? Does she love him enough to let him go?

The couple needs to have common interests. Our pastor told me, "I am always unhappy when I ask a couple why they want to get married, and they can answer only, 'Because we are in love.'"

He prefers to hear the fellow say something like, "Because she is smart, and she believes as I do, and I think she will make a wonderful mother." Or to hear the girl say, "Because I have a great deal of respect for him, and I believe he will be a good spiritual leader in our home, and we can talk freely about any subject."

Any marriage is stronger if the couple can share broad and different experiences, and if each can express his or her inner thoughts.

For some people, sexual intimacy is easier to achieve than the tenderness that comes with being open with each other emotionally and spiritually. They fall into the trap of being able to touch outwardly, but never being able to commune with the other's inward spirit.

According to Herbert G. Zerof, a prominent psychologist, many young persons today have an unrealistic, fantasy-like view of love. "Human closeness comes naturally when it is not sabotaged by the abstractions of romantic love. When two people come together through kindness, tenderness, liking, and caring, they can discover an intimacy that endures."

Love is so daily. It must survive the hardest of all tests: close contact day in and day out. As any successfully married couple can attest, "Love isn't a feeling; it is an act of the will."

What was the couple's "state of the union" before she became pregnant? Was their relationship already near the breaking point? The pregnant girl may be reluctant to admit this. After all, if she is pregnant by him, but confesses that she no longer loves him, this means that she is "bad."

But she should consider this. Her pregnancy may have occurred not because their love was *growing*, but because it was *dying*. In an effort to restore their relationship to its previous glow, a couple may turn to sex as that only area in which they still feel close.

Rollo May has said, "We can always depend on sex to give a reasonable facsimile of love. But used as a substitute for genuine warmth, it becomes a barrier to anything deeper."

If this is what had been happening in her relationship, the pregnant girl may realize how shallow and unsatisfying it had become. But she may find it easier to face a marriage she doesn't want than to face what she imagines will be disapproval and censure.

She may need to be reassured that she is loved because of *who she is*, not *what she does*—or even in spite of what she does. This is unconditional love, of which Christ is our supreme example.

We can emphasize that making a bad mistake doesn't mean that she is a bad person.

Then we can encourage her to be truthful with herself. If she knows that what she thought was love either wasn't love, or has disappeared, she needs to stop trying to fool herself and to get on with life.

I know that is easier said than done, but what better choice does she have?

Is the pregnant girl very young? Today's unwed mother is far more likely to be in her early teens than was the unwed mother even ten years ago.

Often, the younger the girl is, the more she will resist listening to reason. Who says she doesn't know what she wants to do? And don't quote statistics: they are all about someone else, not about her.

Certainly the very young girl is not ready for marriage. But how can she be convinced of that?

For one thing, I believe we need to assess carefully what she is (or isn't) saying. We should take time to probe, patiently and gently but firmly, until we are sure that she is being honest both with us and with herself.

Is she trying to regain the approval of her parents or friends? Is she impressed with the idea of marriage because it impresses her peers?

We can tell her that we know marriage was the first thing that popped into her mind when she first discovered she was pregnant. Then we can explain that, even though she may have said then that she wanted to get married, we won't think she is foolish if she has changed her mind. Rather, we would believe that this demonstrates her increasing maturity.

It isn't uncommon for couples to change their minds about marrying; it happens all the time. Only a few weeks ago, a girl I knew called off her wedding only six days before the big day. She had mailed invitations, purchased wedding and bridal gowns and flowers and the cake, and had arranged for the church, the minister, and the music.

People were surprised when she called it off, but nobody thought she was foolish. "Far better to wait until they are sure," they said.

Waiting until she is sure may be a compromise that the pregnant girl can live with. It is certainly less traumatic to say, "I'm just going to wait a little while," than to say, "I'm never going to marry him."

As for the person who is trying to help the very young girl make the right decision about marriage, make no mistake: this won't be an easy time. The more the girl realizes opposition to her marriage, the more she may dig in her heels and scheme to get her way.

Yet all along she may be secretly hoping that we

won't give in. All of her tears and pleading may be her way of retaining what is left of her tattered self-esteem.

If worse comes to worse, it may be necessary to pull rank on her. Nobody likes to rule by force, but at times it is the only choice. (This may be radical thinking today, but why must we grant total independence to someone who is incapable of surviving independently?) If the girl is not of legal age, she can be denied permission to marry.

If we sincerely believe that the girl's marriage would be a mistake, then we have an obligation to stand by that belief. If she accuses us of not caring about her, we know better—and some day, she will, too.

Some couples are actually excited by and proud of the pregnancy. One mother I know was shocked, not so much by her daughter's pregnancy as by the couple's attitude. "Here come my daughter and her boyfriend, just bouncing in and asking, 'Guess what?' They thought it was the greatest thing in the world that she was pregnant."

Other young couples may not be that open, but still be secretly pleased. They may feel that the pregnancy proves them to be adults, or that it will clear away any objections to their marriage.

However, such attitudes may underscore the couple's basic immaturity, and should serve as a warning signal that they are not ready for this serious decision.

Some Christians feel that the couple is obligated to marry since they have indulged in sexual relations.

I disagree. In the eighth chapter of John, where Christ is dealing with the woman caught in adultery, he says, ". . . Let him who is without sin among you be the first to throw a stone at her" (John 8:7, RSV). Would we be the first? It would be better to adopt Christ's loving attitude toward one who has sinned, and say to the pregnant girl, "Go and sin no more."

We could help by stressing positively the couple's

need for repenting of their relationship, rather than their need for legalizing it.

Then again, if the couple has faced their sin and received God's forgiveness, they may enter into a marriage that is good and enduring. "I know a couple who decided to marry when she became pregnant," a friend told me. "They even went on into the ministry. But they were first honest with each other and with God, and recognized their need to repent."

Occasionally, a pregnant girl may be urged to marry simply because her marriage is viewed as a quick end to the disgrace she has caused. But surely nobody wants her to enter into a marriage which is based on flimsy concession, rather than firm commitment.

If we have prayed about her decision regarding marriage, our next step may have to be backward: we must step back from the situation and leave it with God.

It is never easy to avoid meddling when someone we love appears to be heading for trouble. My grandmother used to say, "When children are little, they step on your toes: when they grow up, they step on your heart."

The pregnant girl who decides to marry may need our help again all too soon. If we make a bitter scene and stir up a lot of bad feelings, she may not feel that she has anyone left to turn to.

I am not saying that she should enter into marriage with the idea that she can call it off as soon as the going gets rough. As a Christian parent, I have always emphasized the teaching of the Bible about marriage. It is a one-time permanent commitment of each partner to the other.

However, there may come a time when a girl has no choice. One young woman in our city tried to make her marriage work, even though her husband continually mistreated her. When he attacked her with a knife, resulting in the miscarriage of her baby, she had to end the marriage.

When Sandy announced that she definitely was not going to marry Jim, I was both relieved and apprehensive. Relieved since I believed she had made the right decision, and apprehensive since I knew so little of what to expect in the months ahead.

Because I loved her, I did want to stand by her and help her during her pregnancy, even though I wasn't sure how to help. The months ahead proved to be a learning time for both of us.

7

While She's Waiting

The immediate crisis was past. Now I yearned for nothing more than to sit back and recuperate. But a vague uneasiness stirred in my weary mind.

I felt as I might if I were walking down a dark street in a strange city and suddenly heard footsteps behind me. While I couldn't say for certain that the footsteps meant trouble, I didn't know where to turn for help, either.

As the days and weeks passed, this uneasiness increased. I began to realize that Sandy could not allow herself the luxury of simply sitting back and passively waiting for nature to take its course. Before her baby was born, Sandy must do some serious thinking. Her future and her baby's future depended on the decisions she made now; Sandy had to begin carefully considering her options.

She received some help in making these decisions from the Christian counselor she consulted. She also would gain practical assistance from a local social service agency.

Our city has several of these agencies. Sandy first became aware of them when she visited with Rose, the volunteer at the emergency pregnancy service.

Sandy knew which agency provided which primary service: adoptions; live-in facilities for the mother-to-be; single parent assistance; or some combination of these.

Although she knew a little about these agencies, yet she remained reluctant to contact one. Weeks passed. Still she put it off. She hadn't decided what she wanted to do with her baby. And neither of us wanted a stranger interfering in this private matter.

Sandy had some other reservations, too. "What if they force me into adoption?" she asked.

I wanted to reassure her that that would never happen, but my background was too full of horror stories about babies who were snatched away immediately upon delivery, babies whose mothers never once saw them. The thought made me go cold all over.

"I'll go with you the first time to be sure you don't get pushed into anything," I said.

Now these fears seem ridiculous, but we didn't know any better then.

Our first appointment with the agency Sandy selected was at 1:30 on a Tuesday afternoon. Both Sandy and I shared a hesitance about walking into that building.

I suppose Virginia, Sandy's counselor, is accustomed to this sort of reception. She seemed to understand how tentative Sandy and I felt. As soon as introductions were made, Virginia explained what she hoped her role would be in Sandy's life.

"I want to help you know what choices you have, and how we can help you to make your choices work," Virginia told Sandy. "We provide both adoption services and assistance to the girl who wishes to be a single parent. Our greatest concern is the baby's well-being. If we help the mother make a good choice, then we will have helped the baby, too."

I began to relax. The unnamed dread—"My, what big claws you have . . . all the better to snatch your baby with. . . ." began to fade away.

Instead, Virginia took great pains to *describe* all of Sandy's alternatives, but to *prescribe* none of them.

Is the pregnant girl unable to continue living at home? Is she unable to support herself? They could provide low-cost housing.

Does she need to continue her education, or go back to work after her baby is born? They could provide day-care facilities for the baby.

If she had immediate need of financial assistance, Virginia could tell her how to apply for Aid to Dependent Children payments. (I hadn't realized that the unwed mother may be eligible for such payments even before her baby is born.)

If Sandy wished, she could attend group sessions one night per week, meeting with other pregnant girls. A trained counselor helped the girls understand the problems or feelings they discussed. For some girls these sharing times provided a welcome opportunity to form new friendships.

In the event that Sandy had no means of paying the medical expenses associated with her prenatal care and delivery, the agency could provide financial assistance.

Virginia was so beautifully calm and logical. Simply by contrast, I could see how much Sandy and I were running on pure emotion. While Virginia did care about Sandy, as a trained counselor she didn't let that caring interfere with the job she had to do.

The biggest question Sandy and Virginia shared was the inevitable choice: what would Sandy do with her baby?

Would she choose to be a single parent? Had she considered adoption? Virginia emphasized that either choice Sandy made could be equally "right."

"It might interest you to know how some other girls made their decision," Virginia said. She told Sandy that some girls were doing an excellent job of raising their own babies. Others had chosen to relinquish custody of their babies right at birth. A few asked that their babies be placed in a temporary foster home while they made up their minds.

"One girl kept her baby for nine months before she realized that she just couldn't cope," Virginia said. "We placed her baby in an adoptive home. It was much harder for this mother, though, after all that time."

Sandy asked Virginia when a girl had to sign papers if she were considering adoption.

"She doesn't need to sign any papers until after the baby is born," Virginia explained. "She can talk over her decision with me, but nothing she says obligates her in any way. Her decision is never final until she is ready for it to be final."

That was a big relief to both Sandy and me. "If you think you may choose adoption," Virginia continued, "you can still change your mind at any time. Or if you decide to keep your baby and later decide it isn't going to work, we will be here to assist you then, too."

Probably one of the greatest benefits to accrue to Sandy from visiting with Virginia was that Sandy gained time in which to think over thoroughly what she would choose for her baby's future.

The unwed mother should never postpone this decision until her baby is born.

If the agencies in other cities are anything at all like the one that helped Sandy, and the counselors like Virginia, I believe the pregnant girl has everything to gain and nothing to lose by accepting the help they have to offer.

Often, a pastor or minister can steer the pregnant girl to the agency which would best suit her needs.

Or she can look under "Social Service Organizations" in the yellow pages of her telephone directory. Also, in our city, at least two agencies run daily newspaper advertisements in the "Personals" column of the classified section.

A word of caution: when looking for this type of

service, the pregnant girl should be careful to deal with a well-known and respected organization. Some persons who represent themselves as "concerned helpers" are concerned only with helping themselves to the money the unwed mother's baby can earn for them. They are not at all concerned with the welfare of the mother or her baby. (I will have more to say about this in a later chapter.)

The pregnant girl who is reluctant to visit a social service agency might do well to bear in mind that she doesn't lose any rights or any freedom of choice simply because she discusses her situation with an agency. It may well be that she gains even more awareness of her rights and greater freedom to choose because of the assistance the agency can provide.

During her pregnancy, the girl may also need to be aware of recent legislation which relates to her.

Of particular interest to her are Title VII of the Civil Rights Act of 1964, and the Pregnancy Discrimination Act, signed into law on October 31, 1978, and amending Title VII.

Because of these laws, no woman, due to pregnancy, childbirth, or related medical conditions can:

1) Be excluded from employment, or prohibited from applying.

2) Be forced to accept different benefits than any other employees regarding commencement and duration of leave, accrual of seniority, reinstatement, or insurance payments.

The Pregnancy Discrimination Act deals in detail with several areas in which the unwed mother in particular may feel the pressure of discrimination. They include sick leave benefits; ability to function and the employer's requirement to provide alternate duties; vacation and pay increases; hiring in the first place; and others.

Basically, what the Act seeks to ensure is that the pregnant woman, married or unmarried, receives the same benefits during employment as anyone else would receive.

For instance, if the pregnant girl applies for a job, the employer "cannot refuse to hire a woman because of her pregnancy-related condition so long as she is able to perform the major functions necessary to the job. Nor can an employer refuse to hire her because of his preferences against pregnant workers, or the preferences of coworkers, clients, or customers."

If the pregnant girl wants to work as a clerk in a department store, she cannot be refused employment simply because, from time to time, the job involves carrying heavy boxes of stock. Since her major duty would be clerking (i.e., waiting on customers, operating a cash register, etc.), then the employer would have to get someone else to do the heavy lifting. But the employer cannot refuse to hire her.

If the pregnant girl feels that she is being unfairly discriminated against because of her pregnancy, she may go to the Equal Employment Opportunities Commission Office in her city and ask for their intervention. While the Commission does not have the power to enforce this law, it can give her advice on how she should proceed if she has a legitimate complaint.

Often, if the pregnant girl's case is deemed to be one of discrimination prohibited by Title VII, as amended, a letter to the offending employer from the EEOC will help to correct the matter.

In the event that the girl lives in a small town or does not wish to go in person to the EEOC Office, she may write directly to the Equal Employment Opportunities Commission, Attn: Office of Public Affairs, 2401 E Street, Washington, DC 20506. She should outline the details of the alleged discrimination against her and request their assistance.

Those who wish to obtain their own copy of the

Pregnancy Discrimination Act may write to the EEOC at the address above, directing their request, "Attn: Office of Policy Implementation." Ask for "Title 29 of the Code of Federal Regulations, Part 1604.10."

The pregnant girl who is still a member of the public school system also has a brighter outlook today.

When I was in high school in the fifties, the girl who became pregnant was not allowed to stay in school. Fifteen years later, as related in *The Rights of Americans,* this policy still hadn't changed:

The unresolved issue which most clearly stands out is the suspension or expulsion of girls, both married and single, who become pregnant. . . . This is a cruel response to a situation in which the unwed girl needs education and sympathy more than ever before. A few courts are beginning to recognize that there is no reason to exclude pregnant girls from school, and this trend is likely to continue.

Somewhere between 1970 and today, this trend has become the norm. When I wrote to the superintendent of schools in our district to see what their policy was relating to the unwed mother, he replied:

In our district, a pregnant student is treated no differently than any other student. While the girl is absent from school, work is provided for the student so that she can complete course work just as we would any other student absent for medical reasons.

We do not provide child care service when she returns to school.

Counseling from guidance counselors and the school nurse is available to the girl.

So the pregnant girl today does not have to leave school simply because she is pregnant, any more than a boy would have to stay at home because he broke his arm and is wearing a cast. Each physical condition may lead to some awkwardness in the classroom, but neither is a basis for refusing to allow the student to attend.

However, if the pregnant girl is not comfortable in the classroom, she can continue to study at home. This is something she should discuss with her guidance counselor.

If she does not feel that she is getting all the help she needs to continue her education under her present circumstances, she may need someone to go to bat for her. An adult may have greater influence than she would with her principal or her board of education members. These administrators serve so many students and have so many demands on their time that it may be necessary to be a "squeaky wheel" in order to draw attention to the girl's needs.

The benefits of continued education for the pregnant girl are obvious: a better life style; training to go on to higher education, if she desires; a boost to her self-esteem, and more.

Although she may begin to feel that she is going to be pregnant forever, the time will pass before she knows it. One hopes she will have used her time wisely, so that when she enters the hospital for her delivery, she can use all of her energy where it's most needed: to bring that baby into the world.

8
Out of the Dark Ages

Time passed and Sandy grew more and more pear-shaped. Her baby began to stretch and explore, finding that delight peculiar to babies in the womb of locating mother's rib with a healthy kick, or practicing gymnastics while mother is trying to sleep.

Sandy's due date came and another two weeks passed before she showed any indication of going into labor. We lived from day to day, sure that any plans we made would be interrupted by the baby's arrival.

Finally, one evening after we had finished the supper dishes, she said, "I feel kind of funny. Maybe I'm having labor pains."

Her contractions continued, off and on, all evening. At midnight we decided to go to bed. I had just fallen into deep sleep when she came in and stood by the side of my bed.

"They're getting harder and closer," she said. "About five minutes apart. Think we should call the doctor?"

Two o'clock in the morning. What sane person would choose to be an obstetrician? But we called, and were advised to go ahead and bring her to the hospital.

Both my husband and I reacted as if we were first-

time fathers. We threw on our clothes, hurried to the
car with Sandy, and raced off for the hospital. I knew
better, but I kept having visions of being pressed into
amateur midwife service.

Once she was checked in, we learned that we need
not have bothered to hurry. "You could both go home
and get some sleep," the nurse told us. "It's going to
be a while, and we can call you when things start to
move along more quickly."

My husband and I looked at each other. "I wouldn't
sleep if I went home, anyway," I said. He agreed. For
the rest of the night, we took turns staying either with
Sandy or in the father's waiting room.

When we first arrived, Sandy's father took care of the
admittance paperwork. He signed the "Consent to
Treatment" forms, and also forms assigning insurance
benefits to the hospital. (Since Sandy was living at home
and was under the age of twenty-one, her father's group
insurance hospitalization plan covered her entire hospital
bill. The girl who does not have insurance coverage
should discuss her plans for paying the hospital bill
before she has to enter the hospital. If she is receiving
help from a social service agency, the agency may be
able to provide financial assistance.)

Her father also was asked to give the name of Sandy's
physician, dates of any previous hospitalization, and her
Social Security number.

The nurse who checked Sandy into the labor room
asked her all the routine questions—when her
contractions had begun, her due date, whether she had
had any previous pregnancies or miscarriages,
complications, or operations, and what visible signs of
labor she had had.

Once the nurse completed her initial examination of
Sandy, she prepared to begin using the fetal monitor
which sat on a counter next to Sandy's bed. "Don't
worry that we think something is wrong with you or

your baby because we are monitoring you," she explained. "We use this for all patients."

Placing two belts around Sandy's abdomen with sensors directly over the womb, the nurse then adjusted the monitor. A strip of graph paper began to print out.

"This line on the graph charts your contractions," the nurse said, "The other monitors the baby's vital signs. Even when we aren't in the room with you, we can watch your progress on the screens in the nurses' station."

I continued to be impressed with the improvements which have been developed in the field of maternity care. Supervision was far more constant than I recalled from twenty years earlier. Indeed, a steady stream of hospital personnel passed through Sandy's doorway— nurses checking her progress, the staff physician who administered Sandy's anesthetic (which she and her personal physician had decided upon before she entered the hospital), and the resident on duty.

This supervision, along with the data provided by the fetal monitor, meant that any abnormality in the delivery process would be detected and dealt with immediately.

Much of Sandy's discomfort was alleviated by the anesthetic she received; the breathing techniques she had learned at prenatal classes helped, too.

Sandy especially appreciated the hospital policy which put one nurse on each shift primarily responsible for her care. It was very comforting that the nurse who assisted her during the last stages of labor and transition also accompanied her to the delivery room and to the recovery room. This seemed to lend a certain security to Sandy when she really needed it, especially since I couldn't go into the delivery room with her. Sandy had asked if I would, and I had tentatively agreed. But I secretly dreaded the ordeal; I get a queasy stomach if one of my children so much as cuts a finger.

As the nurse prepared to wheel Sandy from the labor

room to the delivery room, I asked her, "Do I have to put on a gown?"

For a minute, the nurse looked surprised. "Have you cleared this with Sandy's physician?" She hesitated. "I really think it would be better if you didn't come along. Mothers tend to be far too emotionally involved, and it is pretty hard on them to watch a daughter in her delivery."

I began to protest, but there wasn't time. The nurse was moving Sandy, bed and all, out of her labor room into the hall. "I'm sure she's going to be too busy to notice if you're there," she said.

Relief and remorse played leapfrog inside of me. Since there seemed to be no other choice, I trudged down the hall for one last siege of waiting. If I had learned anything from Sandy's labor, it was how hard it is to be the one standing by watching. And I always thought fathers got off so easy.

The next hour was one of the longest I've ever known. The hands on the clock seemed glued in one place. My husband, Sandy's older sister, and our pastor passed the time talking, but I just wanted to be left alone. My thoughts were with Sandy.

Sometimes I picked up the book in which others who had waited had written their comments. Or I wandered over to the nursery window and watched the babies. Mostly, though, I wore a path between the waiting room and the corridor leading from the delivery room. I'd just about given up watching when I saw Sandy's physician headed our way.

"Well, well," he greeted us. I wanted to shake the news out of him. Hurry up! "Sandy has a fine baby girl," he said. "They're doing just fine. You can see your daughter in the recovery room in just a few minutes."

After giving us the baby's vital statistics, he left. We hurried to the recovery room; Sandy wasn't there yet. Then we rushed back to the nursery window.

Could that be Sandy's baby, lying underneath that
light? "She has black feet," I said.

My husband laughed. "Don't you suppose that's from
taking her footprint? It's just ink."

We strained to get a better look. All we could tell
was the color of her hair. Then we returned to the
recovery room.

Sandy lay quietly. Her face was white. She had several
blankets pulled up to her chin, but she still shivered.

I touched her forehead. "Hi, honey, Glad that's all
over?"

She nodded. "Have you seen her yet?"

"I think so. They didn't have her name tag on her
bed yet, so I couldn't be sure it was she." I squeezed
Sandy's shoulder. "If it was, she sure is pretty."

That brought a wan smile from Sandy. "I've thought
of a name for her," she said. "It came to me right after
she was born. I want to call her Roseann."

"That's funny," I said. "Oh, not the name you chose,
but your timing. I named you right after you were born,
too."

When we left the hospital, we were too tired to know
that we were tired. We stopped for a quick supper, and
I called my friend who was caring for my youngest
daughter. She insisted on keeping her overnight. "Bless
you," I said, "that's a relief." When we finally were
home again, I went straight to bed, and I don't believe
I moved once all night.

For Sandy, there in her hospital room, sleep was
harder to come by. The initial relief after her delivery
was quickly replaced by tensions which she felt she
must resolve before she left the hospital.

Above all, she wondered if she should abide by her
decision for adoption.

9

A Time of Decision

All during her pregnancy, Sandy had lived with a constant concern over the decision she would make for her baby's future. I remember her saying several times, "If I could only be sure I'm doing the right thing."

One of my friends said to me, "I hope Sandy thinks very carefully about this choice." Little could she know how often, or to what extent, Sandy wrestled with this— nor how desperately I tried to listen and share Sandy's concern without unduly influencing her decision.

Sandy decided on adoption about a month before her baby was born. Although she dreaded the pain of separation, she believed her choice would be best for her baby. She felt unprepared for parenthood.

Sandy had changed her mind several times before, but this time she appeared to have an assurance that had been lacking. That she had made up her mind before the time came for her baby's delivery was a blessing. Just getting through labor and delivery and all of the postdelivery hormonal and biological changes is enough for any woman, without adding the pressure of deciding about her and her baby's entire futures.

I doubt that anyone could make a calm, objective

decision in the midst of the slightly unreal atmosphere
which prevails on a hospital maternity ward. It is too
easy to become caught up in the excitement and
anticipation that is everywhere present.

One of the nurses visited with me about Sandy's
decision. "I feel sorry for some of these young
mothers," she said. "Even if she's made up her mind to
allow her baby to be adopted, someone—a mother or a
grandparent or a friend—will come along and try to
change her mind." She shook her head. "Of course, that
same person will probably be too busy to help the
mother when she needs a little time off, or if her baby
is sick. Sometimes people just don't think."

I thought of what she had said when I stood outside
the nursery window, looking down at Sandy's baby girl.
Roseann—precious baby. Something inside of me
yearned desperately to lay claim to this baby. My first
grandchild. I was totally unprepared for the intensity of
attachment I would feel for her.

Had that nurse read something in my mind that I
myself didn't realize was there? I couldn't put the
question to rest.

I was beginning to realize how hard it would be to
let go of Roseann, especially now that I had seen her.
And yet, I was thankful for the arrangements Virginia
(Sandy's social service agency counselor) had outlined
for Sandy's stay in the hospital.

"We recommend that she stay on the maternity ward
after her delivery, and that she see and love and mother
her baby as much as she desires," Virginia said.

In the past, hospital procedures often dictated putting
the unwed mother whose baby was to be adopted with
female surgical patients.

"However," Virginia explained, "a good deal of
thought and study has been done about this, and new
ideas have evolved about what would truly be best for
the mother and her baby."

Sandy was just as much a mother, with just as many rights concerning her baby, as any other mother in the hospital. When she accepted this, she could hope for a more honest and open adjustment to her situation. Instead of pretending that she never had a baby, instead of never looking at or touching her baby, Sandy would be encouraged to do just the opposite.

"But doesn't that make it all the harder when Sandy and her baby are separated?" I asked Virginia.

"Yes, it probably will. But she faces the pain and grief of her loss at the time of her loss; she doesn't try to deny her grief simply by denying that she ever had a baby. Suppressed grief won't stay suppressed forever. Sooner or later, it is going to raise its ugly head and demand attention, probably when Sandy is least expecting it."

Virginia explained further that the girl who gives up her baby for adoption without ever seeing him may worry that something was wrong with him, but nobody ever told her.

Also, when she marries and has a baby she wants, this girl may experience difficulty in developing normal warm and tender feelings for her baby. She may feel withdrawn and indifferent, because in her first pregnancy, the natural mothering process was cut off abruptly upon delivery of her baby. Now, even though she is married and knows intellectually that she will be keeping this baby that she wanted, she still prepares herself emotionally to experience loss and separation.

After considering these factors, we agreed to go along with the arrangements that Virginia proposed. I hadn't realized how startling they would be to the hospital personnel, though, until at least four different nurses approached me to ask, "Are you sure this is what you want? Sandy is to stay on this floor? And see her baby every day?"

By this time, I was beginning to wonder if I was sure.

It had sounded logical when I discussed it with Virginia earlier. Again, though, this decision was thankfully arrived at in a calmer moment. Although it was difficult to stick by it when it proved to be such a new and different approach, I chose to do so.

Neither Sandy nor I has ever been sorry.

The morning after Sandy's delivery, a representative from the newborn nursery visited with her. Together, they decided that Sandy should call the nursery whenever she wished to have Roseann brought to her, rather than having her brought regularly at four-hour intervals as the other babies were. This turned out to be an ideal arrangement.

If it was Roseann's feeding time when Sandy called, then she would give her a bottle of formula. Other times, she would hold her, or simply watch her sleep. "I think she sleeps all the time," Sandy said.

When Roseann was two days old, I was preparing to leave the hospital at the end of evening visiting hours. The nurse in charge of the newborn nursery stepped into Sandy's room. "Are you Sandy's mother?" she asked me. "Would you like to hold her baby?"

Until that moment, I hadn't realized how fervently I did want to, or even that I possibly could. I knew the privileges granted to a mother and father; where a grandmother fit into the picture wasn't too clear to me.

"Oh, could I? Yes, I'd like to very much."

Minutes later, I stood in the line of new fathers, waiting to don my hospital gown and scrub to the elbows. I suppose I looked out of place, but I didn't care. I'd never seen Roseann without a pane of glass between us, much less touched her, and I might not ever have the chance again.

After scrubbing, I held my hands carefully in front of me and backed through the door to Sandy's room. I mustn't get contaminated. Only a few minutes passed as I waited with Sandy for Roseann to be brought to us, but it seemed forever. Finally, the door opened. There she was. Sandy's baby. Roseann—all six pounds of her. A bundle of delicate femininity, wrapped in a pink blanket and lying peacefully in her tiny rolling bed.

The nurse left. For a moment, neither Sandy nor I moved. "Go ahead, Mom," Sandy offered.

My hands carefully encircled Roseann's tiny body, and I perched on the edge of a chair with her.

Oh, Roseann, I thought, *I didn't know I would love you so much.* I held her gingerly on my lap, with her head on my knees. If I ever once held her up close against me, I knew I could never let her go.

That visit lasted a brief eternity. I had the strangest feeling that there were two of me: the one who sat in the chair holding Roseann, and the other who stood in the corner and watched this grandmother and grandchild. That scene is as clear in my mind today as if it had taken place last night.

I especially remember the look of poignant pride and love reflected on Sandy's face as she watched us.

Roseann seemed content to lie quietly. I suppose I made some sort of baby talk to her; I can't remember exactly how we passed those moments together, except that she smiled.

"Look at that," Sandy exclaimed. "How come she smiled for you?"

"Must be the grandma's touch," I replied, lifting a phrase I'd heard my own mother use. Grandma—me!

I wanted to do or say something very profound and meaningful at this extraordinary moment, but I could think of nothing. I was glad when Sandy reached for the camera her sister had brought. Good, I thought, let's get some pictures. That's important.

We straightened Sandy's bed, and then cradled Roseann on the pillow. Sandy handed the camera to me. To my dismay, I saw that only one picture remained to be taken. And we had no more film.

"You take it, Sandy." My pictures rarely turn out well. While Sandy peered through the viewfinder, I prayed that she would get a good picture.

(Later, when I picked up the packet of developed prints, I could hardly bear to look. I flipped through all the others until I found the one that mattered, and breathed a huge sigh of relief: it was a good picture. I carry a copy with me all the time.)

All too soon, the nurse was back. What intuition had prompted her to allow me to hold Roseann?

This was only one of many kindnesses shown to Sandy and me by hospital personnel.

The nurse who checked her into the labor room praised Sandy for making an unselfish decision. "I have two wonderful children, both adopted," she said. "If it weren't for the love of their natural mothers, and their sacrifice, I would never have had my family."

During Sandy's recovery, the hospital did not assign a patient to the second bed in Sandy's room. Perhaps this was a coincidence, but I don't think so. I believe they were purposely sparing Sandy the ordeal of witnessing a young couple sharing the joy of their new baby.

Sandy appreciated the visits from the hospital's staff social worker, who tried to prepare Sandy for the feelings she would experience. She encouraged Sandy to talk about them. "If you feel like crying, go ahead and do it," she advised.

On the other hand, there were some moments of tension that were upsetting to us.

One was over Roseann's birth certificate. Sandy was visibly upset when I came into her room that morning. "The clerk who filled out Roseann's birth certificate didn't ask me what I wanted to name her," Sandy said. "She had already written in, 'baby girl.' "

I knew this wasn't right. Virginia had explained to Sandy and me that the unwed mother, even though she may plan to relinquish custody of her baby, has the right to select her baby's name, which is recorded on the original birth certificate.

When I spoke to the charge nurse, she apologized. "That was strictly an error," she said. "I'll have our clerk prepare a corrected certificate."

Of course, Roseann's adoptive parents would choose their own name for her. But it meant a great deal to Sandy that the name she chose be recorded. Suppose, years from now, Roseann should try to locate Sandy. How would Roseann feel if she discovered that her natural mother hadn't even chosen a name for her?

I was still brooding over the birth certificate business when I went to the nursery window and asked to see Roseann. The nurse looked at the baby I was pointing to, then at the other nurse in the room with her, then back at me. She came to the door and stepped out into the hall. "I'm sorry; I can't show you that baby."

Anger flared hot within me. What right did she have to refuse me? Sandy had signed away none of her rights. "What do you mean, you can't show her to me?" I demanded. "I'm her grandmother!"

She hesitated for a moment. "When there are unusual circumstances involved," she said, "we make it a point always to contact the mother before showing her baby to anyone. Sometimes there are people the mother does not wish to see her baby. And we always have in the back of our minds the possibility of foul play. It seems far-fetched, I know, but since a baby was kidnapped from another hospital here last month, we've been extra careful."

I was embarrassed, but she brushed aside my apologies. "That's all right," she insisted. "You didn't know; I'll just go in and call the baby's mother."

Soon she was rolling Roseann's bed to the window. One little clenched fist poked up out of the pink blanket covering her. She was sleeping peacefully. I glanced around the nursery at the other babies. Some were crying, some sleeping; one was having a bath. What was different about Roseann's bed? That's it, I realized. Hers was the only bed which didn't have a big name tag on it.

Another time, I saw a professional photographer at work outside the nursery windows, preparing packets of pictures for all the babies' parents. All but Roseann's.

In a quiet way, the hospital was trying to ensure Roseann's safety. Perhaps some of their precautions were unnecessary, but when they did have to treat Roseann or Sandy differently than the other babies and mothers, they did try to do so discreetly.

Those awkward moments of tension which did occur might have been avoided if Sandy or I had known to call the hospital's staff social worker, or the nurse in charge of the newborn nursery, ahead of time. We could have learned what special procedures might be followed with her baby, and why.

Emotional currents run swiftly during this time of hospitalization. A little advance planning here can help to prevent unnecessary tension.

Overall, the attitude of the hospital staff was to do what was best for the patient, mother or baby. Kindness and concern were freely evident. No doubt everyone realized the turmoil with which Sandy was living, minute by minute.

Not only was she experiencing the normal up-and-down emotional swings that follow delivery of a baby, but she was beginning to perceive the depth of feeling she had for Roseann. Should she stick by her decision for adoption?

And she continued to fret about calling Jim. Every time she stood outside the nursery windows and watched other fathers proudly observing their offspring, a stubborn hope must have flickered in her heart. Might Jim, too, care? Might he want to see Roseann?

10

The Baby's Father
In deed, if not in name.

Sandy could not find peace of mind. If Jim knew about Roseann, would he come to see her? She was his baby. Surely he would want to have one look at her. Wouldn't he?

It was one of Sandy's nurses who advised her, "Why don't you call Jim, tell him who you are, where you are, and that he has a baby girl. Then just hang up."

Sandy told me about the nurse's suggestion. "Do you think I should do it?"

I didn't know how to reply. I had a fairly good idea what the result of her call would be. But it might relieve her mind to know that she had at least given Jim the opportunity to see Roseann. Although hope might ultimately suffocate and die, it seemed to help Sandy to cling to what little hope she had. Jim *might* care enough to come.

I recalled a conversation between Sandy and me months earlier, as we were driving to her physician's office for her monthly check-up. "I don't care if Jim doesn't want anything more to do with me," Sandy asserted. "But I don't understand why he doesn't even want to see his *baby*."

I caught the edge of despair in her voice; she cared all right. "I know; it doesn't seem right." I thought for a minute. "Maybe he can't show love because he never knew love."

"But *I* loved him," Sandy cried.

I drove on. What could I say? How could I answer her? That he would have wanted to stand by her if he truly cared for her? That I wouldn't have seen him walking down the street with his arm around a new girl friend two weeks after he had sat in our living room and dutifully offered to marry Sandy? That she was better off without him?

Cornelius Tacitus, a historian who was born in A.D. 55, said, "It is part of human nature to hate the man you have hurt." Perhaps this explained Jim's attitude toward Sandy. He had to realize that he had hurt her.

A familiar bitterness welled up inside me. It wasn't fair. Sandy was bearing the entire burden.

Suppose that Jim, while driving a car, ran head-on into another vehicle. He'd get into trouble if he walked away from the scene of the accident. Wasn't this predicament even more serious? Why should he simply walk away from this responsibility?

Our pastor's wife and I were talking about this, when a mischievous twinkle lit up her eyes. "I've always thought," she said, "that a fellow who gets a girl pregnant and then walks out on her should get a big purple spot, right in the middle of his forehead, that wouldn't go away until the baby is born."

She laughed, so I did, too. But inwardly I thought it wasn't such a bad idea.

For months, I resisted the message of Matthew 16:27: "For the Son of man is to come . . . and then he will repay every man for what he has done" (RSV). That wasn't fast enough for me. I wanted immediate retribution.

Not until I stood outside the nursery window gazing

at Roseann did my anger toward Jim begin to melt away. The burden of Sandy's pregnancy had been transformed into the wonder of birth.

God granted me another miracle then, too—the miracle of a forgiving spirit. In place of the anger I'd felt toward Jim, I now felt an indescribable sadness. How pitiful to be a father, and not to care. How miserable he must be to have so little natural affection that he could dismiss his fatherhood without a backward glance.

I couldn't believe that he would not be haunted by the knowledge he tried to refuse—that he was the father of a beautiful baby girl.

As far as we know, Jim never came to the hospital or made any other effort to see either Sandy or Roseann.

Perhaps he believed that, having offered to marry Sandy, he had fulfilled his responsibility. But several months earlier, when Sandy and I had consulted a lawyer, we learned that that was not true.

Our lawyer advised us that if Sandy had a good case against Jim, he would be legally responsible for all of the expenses directly associated with Sandy's pregnancy, as well as for child support (should Sandy decide to raise her baby herself) until the child reached the age of eighteen.

In order to determine whether Sandy had a firm basis for further legal action, the lawyer asked several questions.

How long had Sandy and Jim dated? How long had they been engaged? Was there a ring, or some other token of their intention to marry? Did Sandy have any written communication from Jim, in which he stated his feelings for her? Had Sandy dated any other young men within the past year?

He also wrote down the following information (we could have saved some time and expense by having this much prepared ahead of time):

Sandy's name, address, telephone number, birth date, present occupation, salary, and phone number at work.

The names, address, and phone number of her parents.

As far as possible, the same information for both Jim and his parents.

Sandy was also to provide a list of expenses already incurred because of her pregnancy (laboratory tests, medicines, special clothing, etc.), with receipts attached, and to continue to keep track of further expenses.

The lawyer asked whether Jim had admitted to being the father of the baby. When? We gave the date. Under what circumstances? We had called and asked him to come to our home. (In all fairness to Jim, I must say that he did come immediately, even knowing why we had asked that he do so.)

In addition, the lawyer wanted to know what witnesses were present when Jim admitted to being the baby's father. Sandy's father and I, and our pastor. (We had asked our pastor to come to provide the objectivity we knew we couldn't achieve ourselves. Inadvertently, we strengthened Sandy's possible legal action against Jim, too, in that our pastor would be a strong and respected witness should Sandy's case go to court.)

After assessing the facts, our lawyer felt that Sandy did have a good case, and he recommended sending a Letter of Demand to Jim. In it, Jim was requested to pay for those expenses Sandy had listed. The letter also notified Jim that he would be subject to payment of further pregnancy-related expenses, and possibly child support payments.

When Jim failed to respond to this action, our lawyer discussed further steps he could take.

"I can either file a claim in court on Sandy's behalf, or I can file a paternity suit against the baby's alleged father."

I had assumed that the only way to be reimbursed

from Jim would be by legally establishing his paternity.

"No," our lawyer replied. "If there is a preponderance of evidence that Jim is the father of the baby, which I feel that a judge would agree there is, then the result of the claim will be favorable to Sandy. The judge will order Jim to reimburse Sandy for her expenses."

These would include prenatal and postnatal physician's care; delivery expenses (payable to the hospital, Sandy's physician, and other personnel involved, and the baby's pediatrician); sums paid for the clothing and medicines required for the pregnancy; and wages lost when Sandy took time off for work because of her pregnancy, or pregnancy-related conditions.

Also, if Sandy decided to raise her child, Jim could be ordered to pay child support, which might take the form of regular payments at predetermined intervals, or a one-time lump sum payment.

"On the other hand," our lawyer continued, "if Jim had denied, or did now deny, being the father of Sandy's baby, then she might wish to file a paternity suit."

He explained what was involved. If necessary, the judge may order medical testing (which is much improved in its reliability in recent years) to establish paternity.

The judge will also listen to testimony for both the baby's mother and alleged father. If, in the judge's opinion, there is reason to believe that the alleged father is the father indeed, then the paternity of the baby is established. The father is then required to pay court costs, and to pay whatever expenses and child support that the judge decrees.

However, as our lawyer cautioned Sandy, the paternity suit could affect her decision for adoption. "Once paternity has been established," he said, "then Jim will have far greater rights concerning the child than he had before."

(To my knowledge, only in Illinois does the law state without qualification that the father as well as the mother of a baby born out of wedlock must give his consent to adoption. Other states require his consent only if paternity has been established; some require only the mother's consent; and some have no statutory provisions on the matter at all.)

"For this reason, you may wish to consider very carefully the filing of a paternity suit," our lawyer said. He explained that if the paternity suit does establish the father's paternity, then the father can refuse to give his permission for the baby to be adopted. He may wish to take custody himself. Or, if the father contests the adoption but does not wish to have custody himself; or if he wants to have custody but is unfit to do so; or if he moves and cannot be located, then freeing the child for adoption can be delayed indefinitely.

Because Sandy had not yet come to a final decision about her baby's future at that time, she delayed further legal action.

After Roseann's birth and adoption, Sandy once again contacted our lawyer. He suggested going ahead with the claim for reimbursement of her expenses. However, since Jim has moved and Sandy has been unable to locate him, the claim has not been filed. Trying to find Jim may cost as much as Sandy could hope to recover.

So, for the time being, nothing is being done. Perhaps nothing more will be, at least not in this lifetime.

No matter how much Jim refused to acknowledge that he is a father, though, it was his and Sandy's baby girl who lay in that hospital nursery. And it was Sandy who watched the days dissolve into hours, and then minutes, until it was time to leave the hospital.

She had chosen adoption for Roseann. But now that the moment of separation was at hand, could she go through with it?

11

To Whoever You Are, with Love

It was Virginia, Sandy's counselor, who realized that she did not feel up to signing the Final Consent forms—not while she was still in the hospital, and while Roseann was still down the hall from her in the nursery.

"Many girls prefer to wait until they are home before they take this step," Virginia assured her. "They have time to grow stronger, and also to reconsider their decision."

Sandy had signed an order of temporary release for Roseann. This allowed the hospital to release Roseann to the agency, for the purpose of placing her in temporary foster care. Virginia would take Roseann to her foster home when her pediatrician dismissed her (probably about the same time that Sandy was dismissed).

Each moment that passed emphasized the shortness of that period when Sandy would have complete claim on Roseann. First she signed the temporary release; then it would be the final consent.

Both Sandy and I had long dreaded the moment when she must take pen in hand and sign her name to this momentous document. As it turned out, however, nothing would ever compare to the pain that we knew as we left the hospital—without Roseann.

Sandy's physician checked in on her early that morning, and signed his order for her release that day. When I arrived at a little before ten o'clock, it took only a few minutes to gather up Sandy's belongings and help her to dress.

Then I called the desk and asked for an aide to assist Sandy from her room to the hospital exit.

Bless her heart, the aide who responded to my call was just a young girl. She came bouncing in, settled Sandy in a wheelchair, looked around the room with a puzzled expression on her face and asked, "But where's the baby?"

For an awkward moment, we all stared into space. She might as well have asked a person who had had both feet removed where his shoes were.

Please don't make this any harder, I pleaded silently. "She's not coming home with us," I managed to explain.

We made the rest of the procession in silence: wait for the elevator; down the corridor; out the heavy glass doors; into the car.

It wasn't until we were out of the parking lot and out of sight of the hospital that it struck me. We were here, and Roseann was back there. We hadn't even stopped to see her before we left!

A cold panic churned inside of me, and my head began to throb. The road ahead of me blurred. All the way home, I fought an almost overwhelming urge to say, "Come on, let's turn around and go back and get her." I kept remembering the warmth of her little body in my hands, and the tiny, tentative smile she'd tried out on me.

Later Sandy would tell me that she, too, had been fighting that same urge.

During the next days, the two of us plodded through

a period of deep grief. I am sure that Sandy felt her loss even more keenly than I, although I can't imagine how she could bear it. There were moments when the two of us would look at each other, and both begin to cry at the same time. Other times, we simply sat near each other. Words were unnecessary.

Sandy held much of what she was feeling inside of herself, but I knew how deeply she was hurting when she asked to sleep with me that first night, and hours later, I awoke to find that her hand was still clasped tightly over mine.

Ten days after Roseann's birth (could it possibly have been only ten days?), Sandy signed the final consent forms.

She could have chosen to have Roseann remain longer in her temporary foster home; there is no definitive limit on the length of such temporary care. However, Sandy was anxious for Roseann to be placed with her adoptive parents. She knew that the woman who provided temporary care would be kind, but this woman wouldn't be eager to establish a deep and lasting bond with Roseann in the same way her adoptive parents would.

Virginia came to our home, bringing along the forms to be signed and a notary public to witness Sandy's signature.

Since my husband had to be out of town on business that week, I had asked our pastor to be there with us when Sandy took this final action. We appreciated his presence, although it turned out to be less necessary than we had expected.

Actually signing the forms meant little. The significant moment had already occurred when we left the hospital without Roseann. In comparison, signing the Final Consent was a mere formality, a ritual without substance, an afterthought. Separation had already been accomplished.

Our pastor prayed with us; Sandy signed the forms; the notary public added her stamp of witness; and we were left alone.

To my amazement, I felt a deep sense of peace. "I feel as if someone has lifted a huge weight from my shoulders," I said to Sandy. "I don't understand it."

"Neither do I," said Sandy, "but I feel the same way."

For the first time, I sensed that healing had begun to take place. In my heart, I am convinced that the peace and healing we were to know were the result of the many prayers for us which God heard and answered at that time. This peace has abided with certainty within me: "Peace I leave with you, my peace I give unto you: not as the world giveth, give I unto you. Let not your heart be troubled, neither let it be afraid" (John 14:27, KJV).

I can't say I never cried for Roseann again. Many times I have awakened in the middle of the night, full of an intense, almost unbearable aching to hold her in my arms again. Yet, when I meet the new day, the peace is there in my heart again.

Mine wasn't a peace that had to deny sorrow. Rather, it was a peace which allowed me to feel grief at the same time I felt assurance that the One who cared for and sheltered me would understand my grief.

The choice was not easy. Nor was it casual or callous. But it was made. Life moved on.

For a long time, I was reluctant to mention the grief and pain that Sandy and I experienced following Roseann's adoption. I was afraid that I might discourage some other young mother from going ahead with her choice for adoption.

Then I realized that no woman needs to be told; every instinct in her body and heart testifies that she will know sorrow if she is separated from her baby.

What she may not know, however, is the way God can heal her and restore her peace of mind. How he can reach down in love and bind the broken heart. How deeply he cares when one of his own is hurting.

"And I say, 'It is my grief that the right hand of the Most High has changed' " (Ps. 77:10, RSV).

Surely, I thought, we have walked through the valley of the shadow of death. And just as surely, God has comforted us.

If I could go back now, knowing what I have learned, I would do some little things differently.

Naturally, I would have plenty of film and flashbulbs on hand in the hospital.

I would have purchased a dainty little pink velour sleeper, with lace on the collar and a tiny rosebud applique, for Roseann to wear when she met her adoptive parents; it would have been Sandy's special gift wrapping for her special gift.

I would have encouraged more people to visit Sandy in the hospital; she was so proud of Roseann, and loved having someone to show her to.

I would have asked someone else to drive us home from the hospital.

At least this much I would have done differently. But other things I wouldn't change a bit.

The beautiful bouquet of yellow daisies Sandy's grandparents sent to her, with the note she still treasures, "With love to our little sunshine."

The cards friends sent to Sandy, expressing their love and concern.

The time when Sandy's girl friend came to visit, bringing both a gift the girl's mother had sent, and a tiny English ivy plant. (The plant hasn't been very vigorous, but as long as there is one bit of green at the tips of the leaves, I continue to water it.)

My married daughter who came and kept house and amused her youngest sister during that long week, and who filled the emptiness with chatter.

The dear friend who brought us a huge pan of fragrant, homemade apple crisp. We appreciated her gesture of love so much, even though I had to divide the dessert in portions and freeze it so I wouldn't eat it all at once and so some would be left when Sandy felt up to eating again.

The people who didn't find it too awkward to look at Roseann's picture and to talk with Sandy about her.

I wouldn't change any of that.

We were especially grateful for the many fellow believers who assured us, "I'm praying for you." During the entire ordeal of Sandy's pregnancy, they freely gave us their kind and loving support. I'm not sure how we would have managed otherwise.

In an effort to express our appreciation, we asked that the following note be printed in our church bulletin:

"Wait on the Lord; be of good courage, and he shall strengthen thine heart: wait, I say, on the Lord" (Ps. 27:14, KJV). We pray for this strength as Roseann, this tiny bundle of life, moves from our family circle to the new family who waits eagerly for her. We know she will capture the hearts of her adoptive parents, as she has ours. Thank you for your prayers.

Not only did we want to express our appreciation, but we wanted to be forthright and open about Sandy's decision for adoption, and to make her decision formally public.

I thought that a sense of secrecy might lead Sandy to the mistaken belief that she had something to hide. I was sure that stating the truth openly would be much better than hinting at it or leaving questions unanswered.

This was no time to go off in a corner and nurse our wounds by ourselves. Our friends had stood by us all along, and we needed their love and fellowship all the more at this time. Since we were willing to talk about Roseann's adoption, our friends knew how to approach us. Knowing our needs, they were able to minister to them.

As Sandy adjusted to the reality of Roseann's adoption, comfort came to her in imagining the joy of the young couple who became Roseann's adoptive parents.

Sandy and I talked about this a lot. We tried to understand how we would feel if we were the woman who wanted a baby very much, but could not conceive. We thought of the anxious months, perhaps even years, of waiting for the gift of a baby. We thought of the stockpile of love this couple had stored up to bestow on Roseann.

We began to see how God continued to work everything together for good.

It also eased our minds to know the little that Virginia told us about Roseann's adoptive parents. Somehow, the brief sketch she provided made them appear in our minds less as threatening strangers and more as people we could identify with and feel good about.

We learned that this was a Protestant couple (this is a choice the natural mother can specify). From Virginia's description of their worship practices, and because we prayed they would be, we are certain that her adoptive parents are believers. We also learned the ages of both the mother and father, and that they already had one adopted child. To us, they sounded as if they would be ideal parents for Roseann.

Of course, there was always that inner longing to make our own assessment of them. I knew that the agency conducted a thorough investigation, but that didn't tell me all that I wanted to know.

Would Roseann's adoptive mother rock her to sleep? Would she love every little pebble jewel and dandelion rose her little girl brought to her?

Would her father put down his newspaper in the

evening in order to read aloud her favorite story, for the ninetieth time?

What were they really like?

Then Sandy received a phone call from Virginia. "I have some pictures of Roseann which her adoptive parents sent," she said. "Would you like to have them?"

Sandy and I were both overjoyed. Not only did seeing the pictures relieve the burden of always wondering what she looked like; it also seemed to tell us something about the kind of people her adoptive parents were. The kind who had the tenderness of heart to realize what a picture would mean to Sandy. The kind who appreciated her gift enough to personally acknowledge it. The kind who not only were sensitive to the feelings of others, but who proved it by their actions.

Sandy appreciated their gesture all the more because they had made it on their own. Although she had been told, at one of her first visits with Virginia, that she could request pictures of her baby (the agency would then place her baby only with a family who agreed to send pictures), Sandy had chosen not to do so. She felt it would be too painful a reminder to see pictures of her baby. As it turned out, seeing the pictures was much less painful than not knowing what Roseann looked like.

Additional pictures arrived after Roseann's first birthday. I don't know if we will receive others, but we are grateful for those we have.

More times than I can count, I have asked myself the question, as I'm sure Sandy has: "Was it the right choice?"

The longer I think about it, the more sure I am that we never will be sure. All that we can know for certain is that Sandy made the best choice she could at that moment in her life.

It is really useless to make a decision based on how we *might* feel under possibly different circumstances at some point in the future. Nobody can know that.

Sandy appears to have adjusted quite well. She enjoys her present life style, which is far different than what she would know if she were raising Roseann.

Perhaps the greatest tragedy of the unwed pregnancy is that a choice is necessary at all.

Yet, while the need to choose is tragic, each unwed mother has the responsibility of choosing as carefully and wisely as she can, always bearing in mind the future well-being and happiness of her child.

In such circumstances, no choice is entirely right or entirely wrong. However, there is a right way to go about making her choice; doing so is crucial to the pregnant girl's eventual peace of mind.

12

Investigating the Alternatives

"The heart has reasons that reason does not understand."
—from *Wings of Silver*

President Truman is known to have had a plaque on his desk which read, "The buck stops here." The unwed mother carries this sobering truth in her heart.

For all but those few girls who may be mentally or physically incapable of doing so, the decision about the future of the baby born to an unwed mother is uniquely hers.

She needs to approach this very serious decision in the right way.

This involves prayerful deliberation. It also involves a thorough investigation of her alternatives.

She may already have begun this process if she is receiving professional counsel. The counselor can give practical advice, and can help the pregnant girl to understand the feelings she is experiencing.

She might also know a single parent, or a woman who has adopted a child or placed a child for adoption. Their first-hand reports may be enlightening. (Of course, the pregnant girl should bear in mind that most people are likely to feel that, since their choice was right for them, it will be right for anyone else, too. The pregnant girl needs to remember that she has different hopes and dreams than anyone else; therefore, what was right for someone else may not be right for her.)

A minister or physician may be able to help the pregnant girl arrive at her decision.

She can also obtain material from the public library about the choices other women have made, and how these women felt about their choices.

Whatever the pregnant girl's choice, she will be more comfortable with it over the years if she knows she learned all she could about it before she finally made up her mind.

The choice: adoption. It is easy to see now why Sandy and I were so uneasy about the adoption process. We worried too much either because we knew too little, or because what we did know was inaccurate.

For instance, we feared Sandy might be pressured into adoption. Or that she might not be allowed to see her baby. Or that she would have to sign final papers before her baby was born.

We found that it was Virginia, the social service agency counselor, who was best able to clear up our misconceptions.

By listening carefully to what we said, or left unsaid, Virginia discovered what we needed to know. She made every effort to relieve our fears. And she didn't make the mistake of believing we understood everything she said the first time around, either.

Virginia was also well informed about the newest developments and procedures in the area of adoption. She encouraged us to consider trying some of these innovations (including having Sandy see and hold her baby in the hospital, for instance).

She also explained the legal steps involved in an adoption, and the different types of adoption.

Briefly, these legal steps (which may vary from state to state) include:

1. The natural parents' consent to having the child made available for adoption. In most cases, the only consent required is that of the mother herself; usually, unless a legal action has established the paternity of the father, he need not sign the consent (see Chapter Ten).

2. The persons who want to adopt a child make an application for a baby.

3. A public or private adoption agency investigates the suitability of the applicants as adoptive parents.

4. When a judge is satisfied that the consents are valid and that the investigation of the prospective parents has shown them to be satisfactory, he will grant an interlocutory decree.

5. The child is placed with the adoptive family.

6. The final decree is granted after the interlocutory decree expires.

7. A new birth certificate is issued for the child in the name of the adoptive parents, at which point all rights of the natural parents are irrevocably terminated.

(Incidentally, the only one of the above steps that Sandy was present for was the first. After she signed the "Final Consent," all further details were handled by the agency.)

The pregnant girl can choose between two methods of carrying out the adoption. One is the "agency adoption," and the other, the "independent adoption." (The latter is sometimes referred to as a "private placement.")

With the agency adoption, the social service agency will handle all of the legal and administrative details, and will assume responsibility for determining the suitability of the adoptive parents. The pregnant girl has the assurance that all of the proper legal steps, which are designed for the protection of her child, will be observed.

When she chooses the independent adoption, the

pregnant girl substitutes for the agency either a lawyer, physician, minister, or some other person to act as intermediary between herself and the adoptive parents. In this type of adoption, all legalities are observed; further, in most states, the adoptive parents are investigated by an authorized government agency to make sure they will provide a suitable home for the child.

The pregnant girl who believes she may choose the independent adoption will ideally begin to make arrangements before her baby is born. A lawyer must be hired to take care of the legalities. Her intermediary will need time to locate and provide for proper investigation of potential parents.

Usually, the expenses involved in an independent adoption, including medical costs for the mother and baby, are assumed by the adoptive parents. If the pregnant girl should change her mind, she will be responsible for these expenses. She is, however, free to change her mind at any time before she signs the Final Consent form.

Occasionally, a baby may be placed with a relative of the natural mother; this would fall into the category of an independent adoption. The arrangements are made directly between the natural and adoptive parents, but the legalities are not bypassed.

Sometimes circumstances can discourage the girl from choosing adoption. Babies of racial minorities, or those born with handicaps, can be difficult to place. The girl may wish to relinquish her baby, but hesitate to do so if she believes a good home will not be immediately available.

However, the pregnant girl should *never* consider the adoption arranged by the "baby broker" or the "black market" adoption. In such adoptions, all legalities are ignored. Birth certificates are forged in the name of the adoptive parents (whose suitability is never investigated), and the entire transaction is kept out of legal channels.

These adoptions are illegal in every state, because they do not protect the child's rights or well-being.

In one such black market operation, the operators lured pregnant women from foreign countries by promising an all-expense-paid trip to the United States, and that a good home would be found for their children.

In reality, the operators of this scheme cared nothing about the children, but only about the potential profit they represented: a Caucasian baby can bring $25,000 to $50,000 on the black market.

If the pregnant girl has any questions at all about the persons with whom she is dealing concerning her baby's adoption, she should seek competent legal advice. She must know that her baby is being placed by a reputable agency or individual.

The choice: single parenting. What about the girl who wishes to raise her baby herself?

I believe that her chances of successfully fulfilling the role of the single parent increase in direct proportion to her desire to be a single parent. If she is mature, responsible, and highly motivated, she can probably do as well with her baby as anyone else could. She is certainly legally entitled to raise her own child.

Also, today's single mother will find support from several sources: the social service agency; public welfare; and often, from her family and church. In many areas, organizations have sprung up for the sole purpose of assisting the single mother.

It is highly unlikely that today's single mother will run into the type of resistance that a friend of mine experienced some thirty years ago.

Her baby was born at a home for unwed mothers where she had stayed. "Everybody was against my keeping him," she said. "The people at the home were very upset with me for refusing to give in to their demands; they wanted me to put him up for adoption."

While the home couldn't force her to give in, they could make her choice as difficult as possible. Five days after her baby was born, they gave her a bus ticket home and left her at the station. She had a baby, a suitcase, and a bag of formula to manage, and not a dime to her name.

Fortunately, the pregnant girl who desires to be a single parent today will find the concept more readily accepted. Yet while she knows greater acceptance, the single mother may still find life far more difficult than she had imagined.

In her book *Love Child, a Self-Portrait*, Mary Hanes tells of making herself this promise about the child she was raising by herself:

Things would be different from then on. I would know him before I knew anything else. I would stop work and go on welfare, if necessary. I have kept none of those vows, but I've never stopped making them. Every night I say, "Tomorrow I will be a mother." But I've yet to be little more than a part-time custodian, sometimes a tutor, or a sister too old for him to enjoy. And the loss is mine. I weep, for I have had a child and never known him. . . . And I wasn't sure that I'd loved him at all. He was a weed that had grown up without any care or guidance, a wild child.

This woman felt only too keenly the difference between what she had hoped to provide for her child and what she actually could provide. I thought of the Proverb, ". . . a child left to himself brings shame to his mother" (Prov. 29:15, RSV).

The single mother is often caught in this sort of double bind. If she doesn't take a paid job, she may be able to afford only the barest essentials of life. If she does, she may see far less of her child than she would desire.

Some professionals feel that the single mother who has the best chance of succeeding in her role is the one who has several people who are willing to help her.

One of a single mother's most critical problems may be a feeling of isolation. She can become discouraged and depressed, especially if she is constantly struggling with an inadequate income. When she is already feeling down and her baby becomes fussy, she may find herself shouting at him, or even resenting his presence. Then she feels guilty; she isn't a good mother.

What she might not appreciate is that her reaction isn't unusual. She might feel better if she knew that other women have felt the same way on occasion.

I think that we, as fellow believers, sometimes extend too little fellowship and support to the single mother and her child. If she is trying her best, we should certainly do no less. How can we turn our backs on the single mother at the same time that we are protesting abortion? If we feel she should bear her baby, I think we should also feel obligated to help her bear the responsibility her baby places on her.

I don't mean to imply that we need to provide unlimited help. If it was her choice to be a single mother, then following through and shouldering the brunt of the responsibility involved is hers too. Yet when there is a genuine need which we are able to supply, or when the Spirit leads us to offer hospitality, we should be ready to do so.

We might be able to give, or lend, to her some of the basic needs for her baby, such as clothing, a crib, or other supplies.

Our help might include giving temporary shelter to the single mother and her baby. That would be better than having her move in with a relative or any other person who does not welcome her. It's difficult enough for a new mother to get through those first tiring weeks without worrying that someone will be upset every time the baby cries.

We could help her think through some of the unique problems she will face as a single parent. For instance, she will need to be prepared to offer her child, when he grows old enough, an explanation about his father. She needs to understand how important it is to her child's self-esteem that he perceive his father as a good person. Perhaps our best approach here would be to encourage her to discuss this with a professional counselor.

Also, she should be aware that her child will need to have a source of affection in a man. For some children of single mothers, this man may be an uncle, or a grandfather, or a volunteer serving with an organization such as Big Brothers.

While single parenting can present problems, the resourceful person can succeed, if she is willing to work at it. With our support, her chances of success are even better.

As far as I am concerned, one pregnant girl's choice to keep her baby can be every bit as right as another girl's choice for adoption. But there is a third decision which is always wrong.

Actually, this is more accurately a nondecision. This nondecision is never consciously arrived at. Rather, it is made by default—the mother simply allows to happen whatever will. The baby is not so much wanted as simply there. Care of the baby may be haphazard or left to the person who can't avoid it.

Whatever the pregnant girl does, she must be willing to make a deliberate choice, and then to work at keeping it a good choice.

Nobody can tell her what is best for her and her baby. However, every believer who knows of an unwed mother should be in prayer for her, asking that God will grant her wisdom to make a decision which is in accordance with his will.

Perhaps the pregnant girl who needs the most definite guidance in making this decision is the very young girl. More and more of today's unwed mothers are in their early teens. They don't know enough about life yet to make a well-founded decision about such an important matter as a baby's entire future.

The very young girl probably hasn't learned to react to even a relatively simple problem in a realistic manner: "Oh, no, I've got a pimple on my chin; I'm just going to die. . . ."

Again, what she finds crucial to her happiness one day may be forgotten the next. Yesterday's coveted coat may lie in a heap on the floor today.

The person who is discussing with the very young girl her choice for her baby's future should bear in mind how the girl's immaturity will color her decision.

She can't be expected to sit down and logically assess her decision when she has no practical experience to go by. She may see having a baby of her own as quite a lark—she will have a little doll to dress up and show off, or something to call her own. Or she may take the opposite view and fail altogether to recognize the rewards which may be possible in parenthood.

We do no favor to any pregnant girl who has an unrealistic picture of motherhood if we allow her to walk right into it without ever pointing out the other side of the picture.

Perhaps the best way to be sure she has seen the picture as it really is would be to place her right in the middle of it. Let her spend several days with a young mother who is raising one or two babies. She can then see for herself the range of demands the young child or baby places on his mother, as well as the tender moments of reward.

As each pregnant girl considers her decision for her

baby, she might want to think through the following questions.

Does she have a dependable means of support for herself and her baby? If she will have to depend on public welfare, will she be satisfied with the type of life style it will support?

Does she know exactly how much help she can expect from her parents, other relatives, or concerned friends in the way of financial assistance, housing, and child-care?

If she wishes to continue at her job or her education, does she know what sort of child-care she can provide for her baby?

What would she most like to do with her life, and would raising a baby honestly fit in? If not, would she be equally happy raising her baby and choosing some other goal?

Does she want to keep her baby so that she will always have someone who will love her? Is she secretly hoping that if she keeps her baby the baby's father will come back to her?

Has she decided to keep her baby so that she can get even with the baby's father, since he will then have all those years of child-support to pay?

If she wants to keep her baby, does she wonder how this will affect her chances to marry?

Perhaps she feels that she could do well as a single parent; does she simply lack the confidence to stand up and say so?

The decision is difficult. All she can know for sure is that her decision is going to affect two lives very directly, and many other lives as well.

Yet only the pregnant girl herself can decide. Although she didn't realize it at the time, when she entered into a premarital sexual relationship, she also accepted the responsibility for making this decision. This responsibility doesn't end until she has made the best decision possible for her baby's future.

Certainly it would be better if she never had to face such a decision. But how can we help our girls avoid this dilemma?

As it has so often since that bright February afternoon when I first learned of Sandy's pregnancy, my mind returns full circle to the question which has haunted me all along: why did this happen, and could it have been prevented?

13

An Ounce of Prevention

Printed in large black letters on a white card, the sign
said, "It's easier not to make a mistake than to correct
it." I suppose the person who attached this sign to that
file cabinet was thinking of the clerical mistake. But I
thought this saying must express the exact sentiments of
many an unwed mother.

Is there a way to prevent young girls from making the
mistake that leads to an unwed pregnancy? How does
the young girl avoid the kind of circumstances where
she is tempted to indulge in the sin of premarital sex?
Is there an answer?

I believe that the answer for the Christian girl is her
consistent, godly life.

When trials and temptations come her way, as they
almost certainly will, she can rise above them because
she can claim God's help. "Then the Lord knows how
to rescue the godly from trial. . ." (2 Pet. 2:9, RSV). If
she is living a godly life, she will be rescued. If she is
not, will she even want to resist?

The girl who is living what she claims to believe will
not be constantly testing her limits. She will be guided
by Scripture: "As obedient children, do not be

conformed to the passions of your former ignorance, but as he who called you is holy, be holy yourselves in all your conduct" (1 Pet. 1:14, 15, RSV). Rather than trying to figure out how far she can go without getting caught, she will be concentrating on how far she can go with God's leading.

Because the Christian girl has within her grasp the means of avoiding the unwed pregnancy, it is all the more frustrating when she falls into this trap. Yet it happens; I know.

". . . Some will depart from the faith by giving heed to deceitful spirits and doctrines of demons" (1 Tim. 4:1, RSV). The moving away from godliness may be barely perceptible at first, but once a girl begins the downhill slide, reversing her direction becomes increasingly difficult.

I've seen this very thing happen in my own life, and I've also had God pick me up and shake me and deal very sternly with me. This is bound to happen as well to the young girl whose turning from godliness leads her into premarital sex.

Even if she does not become pregnant, this sin can leave an ugly scar. When she does become pregnant, the scarring effect spreads to many others as well—the baby, the baby's father, parents and brothers and sisters and other relatives, friends, fellow believers, teachers, pastors, physicians, social workers, and taxpayers. The circle grows larger than anything she ever dreamed of.

Because the effects of the unwed pregnancy can be so devastating to so many, I believe we must search aggressively for a way to prevent it.

We can start by giving our girls a proper spiritual upbringing. We can also give them adequate training about their sexuality.

Teenage Sexuality by Dr. Aaron Hass quotes a 1979 study in which 54 percent of fifteen-to sixteen-year-old girls, and 64 percent of seventeen-to eighteen-year-old girls felt that sexual intercourse before marriage is acceptable.

Regardless of how much we hope that the young girl won't yield to the lure of premarital sex, we can't deny that many are yielding.

This emphasizes all the more her need for proper instruction. The greater the consequences of ignorance, the greater the need to allay that ignorance. Premarital sex can have very grievous consequences. A young girl may set a scene for the rest of her life that is far different from the scene she would prefer. She should have sufficient knowledge to make intelligent, responsible decisions. At the least, she should understand the basic reproductive functions of her body.

What about going that extra step, then, and giving her detailed birth control information? This seems to put us in a quandary. If we provide her with this information, she may construe this to mean that we expect her to experiment with sex. If we don't, then she may become an unwed mother.

We might begin to answer this by examining our motives in providing the birth control information. One mother sent her fourteen-year-old daughter to a physician for birth control pills. Was this mother more concerned about her daughter's welfare or about her own loss of face should her daughter become pregnant? What else could her daughter think, but that her mother expected her to need the pill? Besides, we haven't successfully legislated morality; why should we try to medicate purity?

Further, no birth control method is infallible. Do we want to rely on a solution that may not work? For instance, the rhythm method may fail because the girl's system can be thrown off kilter by such things as emotional stress, illness, high altitude, excessive physical activity, and so forth.

Other methods may fail because the girl is not

properly motivated; she doesn't believe *she* will become pregnant.

Or she may use a contraceptive improperly. One young woman was shocked to learn that she was pregnant. "But how can that be? I've been using my pill every day." Her physician was equally shocked to learn that the young woman didn't understand the pill was to be taken orally.

Even when used as directed, any birth control method has a certain percentage of failure.

Giving detailed birth control information, I believe, is approaching the problem in the wrong way. It is working from the outside in, when what is needed is to work from the inside out. That is, we should focus our efforts on teaching a girl a way of life that will, in itself, prove an unfailing deterrent to the unwed pregnancy— the consistent, godly life.

In addition, she should understand that someone who cares about her expects her to handle her sexuality with responsibility, respect, and reverence. Wouldn't it be sad to think that she failed to live up to any better standards because nobody cared enough about her to set them for her?

Believers everywhere should be ready to demonstrate godly standards of behavior. "Tend the flock of God that is your charge, not by constraint but willingly . . . not as domineering over those in your charge but being examples to the flock" (1 Pet. 5:2, 3, RSV). Young people learn much more from our example than from our exhortation.

In *Psychology of Adolescence*, Luella Cole and Irma Nelson Hall point out what happens when young people lack good role models:

Today, adults go openly in all directions and frankly admit a large variety of attitudes on moral questions. It is not surprising that adolescents find the world confusing and that they are unable to establish moral concepts upon a firm foundation.

Not only may our young people lack good examples, but at the same time they are being subjected to many pressures. The messages which we accept as a routine part of our daily lives may infiltrate our minds and become a part of our thinking without our knowing that it is happening. Popular music: "How can it be wrong when it feels so right?" Advertising: "Use our toothpaste (or shoe polish, or pantyhose) and the person of your dreams will be putty in your arms." Television and movies, too, can exert heavy influence; it seems they are becoming more explicit and are glorifying illicit sex more than ever.

". . . By fair and flattering words they deceive the hearts of the simple-minded" (Rom. 16:18, RSV). The young and impressionable don't know how to sort out what is valid from what isn't.

I believe that we also may not appreciate how little good, solid information our young people possess about their sexuality. We often consider today's young people to be more knowledgeable and sophisticated than they are, especially about sexual matters. We make the mistake of equating exposure with explanation.

Sometimes, too, adults unwittingly contribute to the sexual pressures experienced by young people by encouraging them to grow up too quickly. My sister told me recently that some of her daughter's classmates were beginning to wear nylons to school. That's not such a big thing, but at nine years of age? "It's as if there were a conspiracy against childhood," she lamented.

(Perhaps that is true, when we see a major manufacturer of children's toys marketing a line of cosmetic products aimed at four- to seven-year-old girls.)

Another source of undue pressure is the freedom

allowed in the dating situation. According to Dr. Lawrence Fuchs of Brandeis University, parents in the United States allow far more freedom in dating (no chaperones, little supervision) than do parents in other countries. This aggravates the pressure felt by youngsters who are just beginning to date.

Also, with so many homes where both parents work elsewhere, young people have far greater opportunity to be alone together. This certainly does not help the young person who is wavering between yes and no.

If we care about the epidemic of unwed pregnancies, the least we can do is to help our young people to become properly informed about the sexual sides of their natures. We must decide what sort of sex education our young people need, and where they should learn it.

I do not believe that the best source of sex education is the school or public clinic. The young person needs more than clinical facts.

I certainly wish that I had accepted the responsibility of teaching Sandy about her sexuality. Our first discussion of her reproductive system occurred after her baby was born. As we talked, I couldn't believe how little Sandy knew. She had always appeared so sure of herself and had never asked me about anything, as I assumed she would have if she'd had any questions.

Although it is small comfort, this is a common attitude among adults, according to Dr. Aaron Hass. In his book *Teenage Sexuality* he writes:

Many parents leave the responsibility of initiating sexual discussion to their children. "If he wants to know something, he can always come to me." "If she wanted to ask anything about sex, she would." Sometimes this approach indicates a parent's desire to respect the child's privacy. Other times, this parental stance merely serves to deny their own discomfort in openly discussing the subject. If a teenager does not perceive a certain degree of comfort or willingness in a parent to talk about sex, he or she will find it more difficult to broach the subject.

Actually, as I came to appreciate too late, sex education isn't that one quiet afternoon when woman and young girl go off for a "little talk." Rather, it is a continuing process, a constant learning, a teaching in natural circumstances. It includes the lessons in attitude that a girl learns from seeing tenderness and affection between her parents, as well as other unspoken messages.

While we don't have to arrange an awkward, formal discussion, we can grasp moments alone with the young girl to build upon her sexual knowledge.

Rather than passively hoping the young girl will remain a virgin, we could emphasize what's good about refraining from premarital sex. (She is going to hear enough about the other side of the question; our views deserve equal time.)

For instance, who impresses on our girls that premarital sex is similar to finding out about her surprise birthday party before she is supposed to, and then never knowing the delight of true surprise?

Who tells her that having sex isn't a good way to prove that she is grown-up? The mechanics of sex aren't difficult; even the most ignorant peoples of the world have babies. Having sex doesn't mean a girl is any more grown up than does eating or breathing. It's just one more God-given instinct for the survival of mankind.

Does anyone take time to explain to the young girl how delicate the male ego is, especially when it comes to his sexual abilities? She should know that her husband would place inestimable value on the knowledge that she came to him a virgin. The only way he can be sure of that is for her to refuse to end her virginity, even with him, before they are married.

The couple who are willing to wait until marriage to begin their sexual relationship will gain immeasurably in mutual respect. Their love will be strengthened in a way they won't begin to perceive until years later.

Dr. Charlie W. Shedd touches on this in his book *Letters to Karen*. He advises his daughter, "Back up and have one more look at the endless vistas of love. Here is something you must consider again. Beauty in human relations does not require total knowledge all at once."

Sometimes I believe a young couple turn to sex simply because they are so poor at other forms of communication. What they need may not be so much birth control or sex education as education in all social skills. They need to learn how to talk about their feelings, how to share goals, how to open up their inner beings to each other in a nonsexual manner. This couple might do well to spend time with others who have learned these skills well, or to seek effective counseling so that they can learn to depend not only on physical, but also on other levels of touching and caring to sustain their relationship.

What a girl needs may be something as simple as knowing that a caring adult expects her to say no. In addition, she may need to learn when and why to say no. Often, young girls are not aware that a young fellow is so quick to reach the point where he cannot say no himself. If she wishes to be kind and loving toward her partner, she must not allow their relationship to become so intense that they are pushed past the point of no return. She must learn to say no in a kind and loving manner, and at the right time. This may mean saying no even to being alone together—and generally she knows when the time has come to do this.

Under the right circumstances, a sexual relationship can be all it is meant to be, a beautiful source of strength for a couple's love to each other.

It is this nonphysical element of a good sexual relationship which is missing when sex education is a function of a school or clinic. The warm, human side of the question doesn't lend itself to classroom discussion; neither do the questions of morality, personal responsibility, or commitment. In fact, sex education which does not include these teachings may have the opposite effect of what is hoped for, and lead instead to increased premarital sex.

One father I know told me, "I don't want my children to learn sex education at school." At first I thought he disagreed with their receiving sex education at all. "No, it's not that," he explained. "But I want to teach them my own values and beliefs."

Other people, however, do not believe in any form of sex education, whether at school or anywhere else. "Too much talking about sex just encourages them to go out and try it."

This might be true in the instance where sex education does not include the teaching of values. But if we refuse to talk about sex and make a secret of the way a girl's reproductive system functions, will young girls experiment less with sex?

Unfortunately, experience does not support this. The problem of the unwed pregnancy has always been with us, even during those times when sex was never publicly discussed. If a girl is going to indulge in premarital sex, she is very likely to do so whether or not she has any idea of how to prevent a pregnancy.

Often, in the absence of good information, she latches on to any information that happens her way. In a study undertaken in the early 1970's and reported in *Adolescent Sexuality in Contemporary America,* one-third of all younger adolescents, and about one-fourth of older adolescents, thought that "if a girl truly doesn't want to have a baby, she won't get pregnant."

Or she won't get pregnant the first time, or if she has

intercourse standing up, or if she avoids that two-hour time span once a month when she is fertile. . . .

Even though a girl may possess adequate contraceptive information, she may refuse to use it. "I didn't feel right about deliberately planning for sex," she will say. "If it 'just happened,' then it wouldn't seem quite so wrong."

Then there is the girl who wants to become pregnant, for any number of what she may think are good reasons. She may wish to get married, or to get away from home, or to have someone (a baby) to love, who will love her in return.

Some young girls may need insight into the proper relationship between their spirituality and their sexuality. When sexual matters are not openly spoken of when it would be appropriate to do so, the young girl can end up with wrong attitudes toward her own sexual feelings.

She knows that people she respects try to do what is good and not to do what is bad. If there is an area these people avoid discussing, then the girl makes the mental connection: they avoid this area because it is bad. Therefore, when one of the subjects they don't refer to is sex, the girl naturally assumes sex belongs in the bad category.

Of course, this can be a puzzle to the girl, as she comes to understand that there has to be sex before there are babies, and everyone thinks babies are wonderful.

In her confusion, she may try to deny her sexual desires, thinking they are bad; when they persist, she feels guilty and ashamed. At the same time, she is cut off from talking with the people she respects because she believes that she knows what they think. She may enter into a relationship with a boy simply to have someone to whom she can disclose her sexual feelings.

This illicit relationship might never have occurred if there had been a caring adult with whom the young girl could discuss her sexual feelings.

Demographers at Johns Hopkins University found that girls who said they confided in their parents were substantially less likely to have premarital intercourse than those with little parental communication.

If we can help the young girl avoid premarital sex by encouraging her to talk to us about her sexual feelings, we should be willing to do so.

It is clear that prevention of the unwed pregnancy is a many-faceted problem and that the solutions the world has to offer aren't working. Dispensing the pill and other contraceptives, opening abortion clinics, and so forth, imply that premarital sex is bound to occur and that we might as well accept the fact. The world's attitude is, "We know she'll be tempted, but we can't help that, so we'll just try to help her avoid pregnancy."

The Christian girl, however, *can* be helped when she is tempted: "For we have not a high priest who is unable to sympathize with our weaknesses, but one who in every respect has been tempted as we are, yet without sin. Let us then with confidence draw near to the throne of grace, that we may receive mercy and find grace to help in time of need" (Heb. 4:15, 16, RSV).

She must, however, be living the *consistent,* godly life. Our pastor summed this up when he said, "If we truly confess Christ, then what we say, what we feel, and what we do speak in one way—to support that confession."

If the Christian girl fails to be consistent for even a short time, she leaves an opening for temptation to come in at the same time that she moves away from the One who can make her temptation bearable.

But when her walk is consistent, she will be able to withstand any temptation that comes to her. She will be able to maintain self-control, which is, for the single person, the best form of birth control.

Some Christian girls have learned the hard way, through the unwed pregnancy, what happens when they try to go it on their own. Then they need to learn as well that they can be forgiven. They were not the first to fail in their Christian walk. "All we like sheep have gone astray; we have turned every one to his own way; and the Lord has laid on him the iniquity of us all" (Isa. 53:6, RSV).

God has made provision for each girl's sin. She can be forgiven and welcomed back into fellowship with him.

She needs to know this if she is to use her present difficulties as stepping stones to a better life.

14

Defeated or Different

"The Moving Finger writes; and, having writ,
Moves on: nor all your Piety nor Wit
Shall lure it back to cancel half a Line,
Nor all your Tears wash out a Word of it."

—Omar Khayyam (Tr. Edward Fitzgerald)

The unwed mother can't go back and undo what's done. But she doesn't have to go on living under the shadow of her past, either. She can choose.

Will she allow the circumstances of her past to defeat her, or will she emerge from them a different and better person?

It's easy to understand how an unwed mother might feel that her life is ruined. But when she sees only her present predicament or her past failure, her outlook can become as distorted as her figure.

Christ has forgiven her. She must not dwell on her past: "Set your minds on things that are above, not on things that are on earth. For you have died, and your life is hid with Christ in God" (Col. 3:2, 3, RSV).

She may be one of the walking wounded, but she hasn't lost the entire war.

God provided a sacrifice for our sins. This doesn't mean we will be spared pain and sorrow if we sin. The unwed mother certainly is not spared. Her pregnancy is often a time of heartache and frustration. But this, although painful, can be the tool God uses to discipline her and mold her for her own good. "For the moment all discipline seems painful rather than pleasant; later it yields the peaceful fruit of righteousness to those who have been trained by it" (Heb. 12:11, RSV).

Merely by providing a break in her life style, her pregnancy may prove an unlikely source of blessing. Her life may have become so hectic that she hardly had time to think what she was doing, much less why she did it. Today's young girl may be juggling school, employment, church, athletic and social activities. Often, the unwed pregnancy brings many of these activities to a screeching halt, or at least slows the pace considerably.

With her world moving less frantically, the pregnant girl can rediscover the luxury of uncommitted time. She can use this time to consider where she's heading in her life, and why. If she decides that she wants off, it's far safer and easier to get off if her world is stopped first. She can also use this time to explore her potentials and set new goals for her life.

Her pregnancy may also provide the impetus she has needed to seek out effective counseling. She may thereby gain insights about herself and her feelings that will help her all the rest of her life.

For some girls, pregnancy may bring about their first opportunity to know a grown woman as a close friend. The pregnant girl needs someone who won't give up on her, even when she's ready to give up on herself. She also needs someone she can trust, someone to whom she's not afraid to expose her innermost thoughts. The friendship that results from the concerns that the pregnant girl and her adult friend share can have a very positive effect on both of their lives.

The pregnant girl might well think of her present circumstances as good preparation for her to help some other girl through a similar experience in years to come. "Who comforts us in all our affliction, so that we may be able to comfort those who are in any affliction, with the comfort with which we ourselves are comforted by God" (2 Cor. 1:4, RSV).

It is important, too, that the pregnant girl keep in touch with her fellow believers. The benefits of unbroken fellowship can run in two directions: to the pregnant girl, as she is encouraged by the prayers and support of fellow believers; and to those believers, who may be prompted to reevaluate their own walk with God, or who may discover the satisfaction of lifting up one who has fallen. "Bear one another's burdens, and so fulfill the law of Christ" (Gal. 6:2, RSV).

It may even be that the unwed pregnancy will end the girl's plans to marry a nonbeliever and will lead to her marriage to a fine, godly man. Certainly her hopes of being sincerely loved and cherished will be much better when her husband is in contact with God, the source of love.

It may be years before she perceives how the unfortunate circumstances of her unwed pregnancy have been used by God for her benefit. But she can begin now to point herself in the right direction: she can make a conscious choice.

Will she be defeated? Or different? Will she bury herself in her sinful past, or will she bury her past sin?

". . . But one thing I do, forgetting what lies behind and straining forward to what lies ahead, I press on toward the goal for the prize of the upward call of God in Christ Jesus" (Phil. 3:13, 14, RSV).

My earnest prayer for every unwed mother is that she will choose to begin a new life in Christ, so that she can look ahead to years of service and joy.

She can't ever go back and be the same again. But by God's grace she can be better.

Bibliography

CHAPTER FOUR

Dorsen, Norman, ed. *The Rights of Americans.* New York: Random House (Pantheon), 1970.

Koop, C. Everett, M.D., and Schaeffer, Francis. *Whatever Happened to the Human Race?* Old Tappan, New Jersey: Fleming H. Revell Company, 1979. Used by permission.

CHAPTER FIVE

The Living Bible. Wheaton, Illinois: Tyndale House Publishers, Inc., 1971.
Narramore, Clyde M. *Psychology for Living, Counseling with the Unwed Mother.* Rosemead, California: Narramore Christian Foundation, 1970. Used by permission.

CHAPTER SIX

O'Brien, Patricia. *The Woman Alone.* New York: Quadrangle/New York Times Book Co., 1973.

Zerof, Herbert G. *Finding Intimacy.* New York: Random House, 1978.

CHAPTER TWELVE

Hanes, Mary. *Love Child, a Self-Portrait.* Philadelphia, New York: J. B. Lippincott & Company, 1972. Used by permission.

Petty, Jo, comp. *Wings of Silver.* Norwalk, Connecticut: C. R. Gibson Company, 1967.

CHAPTER THIRTEEN

Cole, Luella, and Hall, Irma Nelson. *Psychology of Adolescence.* New York: Holt, Rinehart, and Winston, Inc., 1970.

Fuchs, Lawrence H. *Family Matters: Why the American Family Is in Trouble.* New York: Random House, Inc., 1972.

Hass, Aaron, Ph.D. *Teenage Sexuality.* New York: Macmillan Publishing Company, 1979. Used by permission.

Shedd, Charlie W. *Letters to Karen.* Nashville, New York: Abingdon Press, 1965.

Sorenson, Robert. *Adolescent Sexuality in Contemporary America, Personal Values and Sexual Behavior, Ages 13-19.* New York: World Publishing Company, 1973.